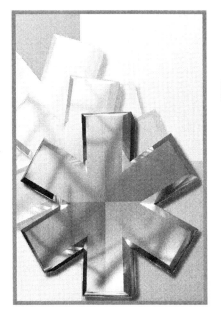

BRADY

ADVANCED MEDICAL LIFE SUPPORT

A PRACTICAL APPROACH TO ADULT MEDICAL EMERGENCIES

SECOND EDITION

Coordinator & Instructor Guide

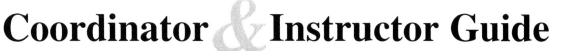

Linda M. Abrahamson, RN, EMT-P
EMS Education Coordinator, Silver Cross Hospital/Joliet Junior College, Joliet, Illinois

Rosemary Adam, RN, EMT-P
Emergency Medicine Educator/Nurse Instructor, The University of Iowa Health Care
EMS Learning Resources Center, Iowa City, Iowa

Ann Bellows, RN, EMT-P, Ed.D.
Training Coordinator, Southwest Air Ambulance, Las Cruces, New Mexico

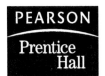

PEARSON
Prentice
Hall

Upper Saddle River, New Jersey 07458

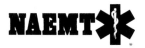

This AMLS Coordinator and Instructor Guide has been developed by Linda M. Abrahamson, Rosemary Adam, and Ann Bellows in conjunction with NAEMT.

Publisher: Julie Levin Alexander
Senior Editor: Tiffany Price
Senior Managing Editor: Lois Berlowitz
Senior Marketing Manager: Katrin Beacom
Director of Production and Manufacturing:
  Bruce Johnson
Managing Production Editor: Patrick Walsh
Manufacturing Manager: Ilene Sanford
Manufacturing Buyer: Pat Brown
Production Liaison: Julie Li
Production Editor: Barbara J. Barg
Creative Director: Cheryl Asherman
Design Coordinator: Maria Guglielmo Walsh
Cover Designer: Blair Brown
Manager of New Media Production: Amy Peltier
New Media Project Manager: Stephen Hartner
Composition: Navta Associates
Slide Design and Production: The Advanced Medical Life
  Support Executive Council, Linda M. Abrahamson,
  Rosemary Adam, Ann Bellows, with special help from
  Arthur B. Hsieh, Christopher Nelson, and Kathryn Roa
Test Material: AMLS Executive Council with special help
  from John Greg Clarkes and Arthur B. Hsieh
Printing and Binding: Demand Production Center

NOTICE ON CARE PROCEDURES

It is the intent of the authors and publishers that this Guide be used as part of a formal education program taught by a qualified instructor and supervised by a licensed physician or as a reference text. The care procedures presented here represent accepted practices in the United States. They are not offered as a standard of care. Prehospital emergency care is to be performed only under the authority and guidance of a licensed physician as part of an organized EMS system. It is the reader's responsibility to know and follow local care protocols as provided by medical advisors directing the system to which he or she belongs. Also, it is the reader's responsibility to stay informed of emergency care procedure changes. The material in this Guide contains the most current information available at the time of publication. However, federal, state, and local guidelines concerning clinical practices, including without limitation, those governing infection control and universal precautions, change rapidly. The reader should note, therefore, that the new regulations may require changes in some procedures.

Pearson Prentice Hall™ is a trademark of Pearson Education, Inc.
Pearson® is a registered trademark of Pearson plc
Prentice Hall® is a registered trademark of Pearson Education, Inc.

Pearson Education LTD.
Pearson Education Singapore, Pte. Ltd
Pearson Education Canada, Ltd.
Pearson Education—Japan
Pearson Education Australia PTY, Limited
Pearson Education North Asia Ltd
Pearson Educación de Mexico, S.A. de C.V.
Pearson Education Malaysia, Pte. Ltd

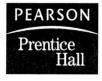

10 9 8 7 6 5 4 3
ISBN 0-13-049424-0

CONTENTS

ABOUT THE AUTHORS

Linda M. Abrahamson, RN, EMT-P, is the EMS Education Coordinator at Silver Cross Hospital, Joliet, Illinois. She currently manages a community college paramedic program and continuing education courses for Will and Grundy counties. She is an active flight paramedic and emergency room registered nurse. Linda has served many local and national EMS leadership roles within NAEMT and other organizations. She is the president-elect of the National Association of EMS Educators. She is the Chairperson for the National Association of Emergency Medical Technician's Advanced Medical Life Support Executive Committee.

Rosemary Adam, RN, EMT-P, is an EMS Nurse, Flight Nurse, and Emergency Medicine Educator with 25 years of experience. She has been active in Iowa and the Midwest in the design, development, coordination, and presentation of many different types of educational programs for EMS providers, nurses, and physicians.

Ann Bellows, RN, EMT-P, Ed.D., is the Training Coordinator for Southwest Air Ambulance, Las Cruces, New Mexico. She has over 20 years of experience in prehospital education. She has worked in ICUs and EDs in small rural hospitals and Level I Trauma Centers. She has clinical experience in fixed and rotor wing transport. She is involved with the NAEMT and has worked to develop the PHTLS and AMLS courses. Ann has been the program coordinator and primary instructor for EMS classes at all levels. She has her doctorate in Training and Learning Technologies with a minor in Message Design.

ACKNOWLEDGMENTS

The authors wish to acknowledge and thank the many reviewers of the second edition of this Coordinator and Instructor Guide. These individuals devoted countless hours of review. Their comments were invaluable in developing and fine tuning this revision.

Randal Benner
Department of Health Professions
College of Health and Human
  Resources
Youngstown State University
Youngstown, OH

Christopher Cebollero, NREMT-P
Medstar
Fort Worth, TX

John Greg Clarkes, NREMT-P
President/Education Coordinator
Canadian College of EMS
Edmonton, Alberta, Canada

Deb Funk, MD
Albany MedFLIGHT
AMLS Medical Director
Albany, NY

Arthur B. Hsieh, MA, NREMT-P
Assistant Professor, Emergency
  Health Services
Department of Emergency Medicine
George Washington University
Washington, D.C.

Bradley Madsen, EMT-P, CCP
EMS Program Coordinator
Mercy Medical Center—School
  of EMS
Des Moines, IA

Brett A. Martin
MICT Program Coordinator
Kapiolani Community College
Honolulu, HI

Anne McGowan-Schooler, MS, EMT-P
Health and Kinesiology Department
College of Education
Texas A&M University
College Station, TX

Sam Micelli, EMT-P
Clinical Coordinator
Dona Ana Community College
Las Cruces, NM

Christopher M. Nelson, EMT-P
Will/Grundy EMS System
Plainfield, IL

Deborah L. Petty, EMT-P, I/C
St. Charles County Ambulance
  District
St. Peters, MO

Kathryn F. Roa, EMT-P
Plainfield Ambulance Department
Plainfield, IL

Keshia Sheppard
NAEMT AMLS Coordinator
Clinton, MS

Jeri L. Smith, NREMT-P, MICT
Flight Medic
EagleMed Flight Program
Wichita, KS

Timothy L. Smith, NREMT-P, MICT
Flight Medic
EagleMed Flight Program
Wichita, KS

ADVANCED MEDICAL LIFE SUPPORT EXECUTIVE COUNCIL 2002

Linda M. Abrahamson, RN, EMT-P
AMLS Chairperson
EMS Education Coordinator
Silvercross Hospital/Joliet Junior
  College
Joliet, IL

Robert M. Domeier, MD, FACEP
National Association of Emergency
  Medical Services Physicians
AMLS Medical Director
St. Joseph Mercy Hospital
Ann Arbor, MI

Vincent N. Mosesso Jr., MD
National Association of Emergency
  Medical Services Physicians
AMLS Medical Director
University of Pittsburgh Emergency
  Medicine
Pittsburgh, PA

**Rosemary Adam, RN, EMT-P
  (Specialist)**
Nurse Instructor
The University of Iowa Health Care
  EMS Learning Resources Center
Iowa City, IO

Ann Bellows, RN, EMT-P, Ed.D.
Training Coordinator
Southwest Air Ambulance
Las Cruces, NM

Will Chapleau, RN, EMT-P
Chief
Chicago Heights Fire Department
Chicago Heights, IL

**John (Greg) Clarkes EMT-P,
  MICP, NREMT-P**
President and Education Coordinator
Canadian College of EMS
Edmonton General Hospital
Edmonton, Alberta Canada

Arthur Hsieh, MA, NREMT-P
National Association of Emergency
  Medical Services Educators
Assistant Professor
Department of Emergency Medicine
The George Washington University
Washington, D.C.

Daniel Limmer, AS, EMT-P
Instructor and Clinical Coordinator
Southern Maine Technical College
South Portland, ME
Paramedic
Kennebunkport, ME

FOREWORD

In 1984, I presented a two-day course on the management of adult medical emergencies to fifty physicians and nurses in Havre, Montana. Based on the already-existing model of "Advanced Cardiac Life Support" and "Advanced Trauma Life Support," the course was named "Advanced Medical Life Support" or "AMLS" for short. Over the next several years, numerous nurses, physicians, EMTs, and paramedics participated in this course. In 1987, my text *Advanced Medical Life Support—Adult Medical Emergencies* was published. Despite initial interest, the time may not have been right, for interest in the course and the text waned. And, my efforts moved in other directions.

The need for a nationally based and standardized course on the treatment of adult medical emergencies, especially to out-of-hospital personnel, has not changed. Today, through the efforts of both NAEMSP and NAEMT, this concept has become a reality. While Twink, Dan, Joe, and Howie have written the AMLS textbook, an NAEMT Course Committee has formulated and will promote the AMLS course. Both the textbook and course are aimed directly at paramedics and employ time-tested strategies. Though I was not personally involved, I derive great satisfaction from seeing the AMLS concept take shape on a large scale. With all the current changes in national EMS, the time seems ripe.

I wish all involved my best.

Mikel A. Rothenberg, MD
Emergency Care Educator
North Olmsted, OH

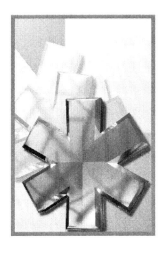

I. COURSE OBJECTIVES

⊞ ASSESSMENT OF THE MEDICAL PATIENT

Ⓐ The participant will be able to apply critical thinking skills to integrate pathophysiology with assessment and history findings to determine actual and potential patient problems.

KEYS *The participant will be able to:*

1) Perform an appropriate scene size-up.

2) Differentiate criteria for stable and unstable patients, their presentations, and transport.

3) Differentiate assessment techniques for patients who are stable and for those who are unstable.

4) Utilize appropriate interviewing techniques to gather the most appropriate information in the shortest amount of time (AVPU, OPQRST, and SAMPLE).

5) Recognize and explain different pathophysiological responses found during the assessment of mental status, airway, breathing, and circulation.

6) Describe the differences in the assessment of the elderly patient.

Ⓑ Given a scenario or case study, the participant will use problem-solving strategies to determine management alternatives.

KEYS *The participant will be able to:*

1) Conduct an initial scene size-up.

2) Differentiate life-threatening situations and initiate the appropriate treatment, including airway management, ventilation, and oxygen therapy.

3) Obtain a generalized patient assessment using appropriate interviewing techniques.

4) Demonstrate examination techniques for evaluating patients with neurological, respiratory, cardiac, and abdominal complaints.

▦ AIRWAY MANAGEMENT, VENTILATION, AND OXYGEN THERAPY

A The participant will be able to apply critical thinking skills to integrate pathophysiology with assessment and history findings to determine actual and potential patient problems.

<u>KEYS</u> *The participant will be able to:*

1) Perform an appropriate scene size-up.

2) Recognize the need for aggressive airway management.

3) Differentiate between different airway management devices depending on the clinical situation.

4) Explain indications and contraindications for each technique or device.

B Given a scenario or case study, the participant will use problem-solving strategies to determine management alternatives.

<u>KEYS</u> *The participant will be able to:*

1) Conduct an initial scene size-up.

2) Utilize the appropriate airway management technique:

   a) Oral endotracheal intubation

   b) Nasal endotracheal intubation

   c) Rapid sequence intubation

   d) Digital intubation

   e) Lighted-stylet intubation

   f) Alternative airway devices (PtL, Combitube, LMA)

   g) Surgical airway alternatives

▦ HYPOPERFUSION (SHOCK)

A The participant will be able to apply critical thinking skills to integrate pathophysiology with assessment and history findings to determine actual and potential patient problems.

<u>KEYS</u> *During a case scenario with an interactive patient, the participant will be able to:*

1) Perform an appropriate assessment.

2) Evaluate for potential risk factors.

3) Evaluate for organ dysfunction.

4) Evaluate for systemic causes.

5) Conduct an appropriate history.

6) Relate medication history to patient problems.

7) Apply pathophysiology to assessment findings.

B Given a scenario or case study, the participant will use problem-solving strategies to determine management alternatives.

KEYS *During a case scenario with an interactive patient, the participant will be able to:*

1) Assess the scene and take appropriate steps for scene management.

2) Initiate immediate management for life-threatening conditions.

3) Differentiate between compensated, progressive, and irreversible shock.

4) Differentiate between hypovolemic, obstructive, distributive, and cardiogenic shock.

5) Develop management alternatives for probable differential diagnoses to include as needed: airway management, respiratory and/or ventilatory support, fluid therapy, pharmacological support, and transportation to an appropriate facility.

⊞ DYSPNEA

A The participant will be able to apply critical thinking skills to integrate pathophysiology with assessment and history findings to determine actual and potential patient problems.

KEYS *During a case scenario with an interactive patient, the participant will be able to:*

1) Perform an appropriate assessment.

2) Evaluate for potential risk factors.

3) Evaluate for organ dysfunction.

4) Evaluate for systemic causes.

5) Conduct an appropriate history.

6) Relate medication history to patient problems.

7) Apply pathophysiology to assessment findings.

B Given a scenario or case study, the participant will use problem-solving strategies to determine management alternatives.

KEYS *During a case scenario with an interactive patient, the participant will be able to:*

1) Assess the scene and take appropriate steps for scene management.

2) Initiate immediate management for life-threatening conditions.

3) Differentiate between primary respiratory causes and all other causes of dyspnea.

4) Develop management alternatives for probable differential diagnoses to include as needed: airway management, respiratory and/or ventilatory support, fluid therapy, pharmacological support, and transportation to an appropriate facility.

C The participant will be able to communicate pertinent patient findings and management to medical direction for further orders and to the receiving facility.

KEYS *During a case scenario with an interactive patient, the participant will be able to:*

1) Verbally transmit patient information in an organized manner.

2) Describe a patient problem in a manner that appropriately relays the patient's condition and the treatment currently rendered.

3) Describe a patient problem in a manner that appropriately relays the need for further intervention.

4) Discuss initial impression and possible etiologies with progression to probable differential diagnoses.

CHEST PAIN

A The participant will be able to apply critical thinking skills to integrate pathophysiology with assessment and history findings to determine actual and potential patient problems.

KEYS *During a case scenario with an interactive patient, the participant will be able to:*

1) Perform an appropriate assessment.

2) Evaluate for potential risk factors.

3) Evaluate for organ dysfunction.

4) Evaluate for systemic causes.

5) Conduct an appropriate history.

6) Relate medication history to patient problems.

7) Apply pathophysiology to assessment findings.

B Given a scenario or case study, the participant will use problem-solving strategies to determine management alternatives.

KEYS *During a case scenario with an interactive patient, the participant will be able to:*

1) Assess the scene and take appropriate steps for scene management.

2) Initiate immediate management for life-threatening conditions.

3) Differentiate between primary causes of chest pain of cardiac origin and all other potential causes.

4) Develop management alternatives for probable differential diagnoses to include as needed: airway management, respiratory and/or ventilatory support, fluid therapy, pharmacological support, and transportation to an appropriate facility.

C The participant will be able to communicate pertinent patient findings and management to medical direction for further orders and to the receiving facility.

KEYS *During a case scenario with an interactive patient, the participant will be able to:*

1) Verbally transmit patient information in an organized manner.

2) Describe a patient problem in a manner that appropriately relays the patient's condition and the treatment currently rendered.

3) Describe a patient problem in a manner that appropriately relays the need for further intervention.

4) Discuss initial impression and possible etiologies with progression to probable differential diagnoses.

ALTERED MENTAL STATUS

A The participant will be able to apply critical thinking skills to integrate pathophysiology with assessment and history findings to determine actual and potential patient problems.

KEYS *During a case scenario with an interactive patient, the participant will be able to:*

1) Perform an appropriate assessment.

2) Evaluate for potential risk factors.

3) Evaluate for organ dysfunction.

4) Evaluate for systemic causes.

5) Conduct an appropriate history.

6) Relate medication history to patient problems.

7) Apply pathophysiology to assessment findings.

B Given a scenario or case study, the participant will use problem-solving strategies to determine management alternatives.

KEYS *During a case scenario with an interactive patient, the participant will be able to:*

1) Assess the scene and take appropriate steps for scene management.

2) Initiate immediate management for life-threatening conditions.

3) Differentiate between various causes of an altered mental status.

4) Develop management alternatives for probable differential diagnoses to include as needed: airway management, respiratory and/or ventilatory support, fluid therapy, pharmacological support, and transportation to an appropriate facility.

C The participant will be able to communicate pertinent patient findings and management to medical direction for further orders and to the receiving facility.

KEYS *During a case scenario with an interactive patient, the participant will be able to:*

1) Verbally transmit patient information in an organized manner.

2) Describe a patient problem in a manner that appropriately relays the patient's condition and the treatment currently rendered.

3) Describe a patient problem in a manner that appropriately relays the need for further intervention.

4) Discuss initial impression and possible etiologies with progression to probable differential diagnoses.

SEIZURES AND SEIZURE DISORDERS

A The participant will be able to apply critical thinking skills to integrate pathophysiology with assessment and history findings to determine actual and potential patient problems.

KEYS *During a case scenario with an interactive patient, the participant will be able to:*

1) Perform an appropriate assessment.

2) Evaluate for potential risk factors.

3) Evaluate for organ dysfunction.

4) Evaluate for systemic causes.

5) Conduct an appropriate history.

6) Relate medication history to patient problems.

7) Apply pathophysiology to assessment findings.

B Given a scenario or case study, the participant will use problem-solving strategies to determine management alternatives.

KEYS *During a case scenario with an interactive patient, the participant will be able to:*

1) Assess the scene and take appropriate steps for scene management.

2) Initiate immediate management for life-threatening conditions.

3) Differentiate between seizure types.

4) Differentiate between primary causes of seizure and all other potential causes.

5) Develop management alternatives for probable differential diagnoses to include as needed: airway management, respiratory and/or ventilatory support, fluid therapy, pharmacological support, and transportation to an appropriate facility.

C The participant will be able to communicate pertinent patient findings and management to medical direction for further orders and to the receiving facility.

KEYS *During a case scenario with an interactive patient, the participant will be able to:*

1) Verbally transmit patient information in an organized manner.

2) Describe a patient problem in a manner that appropriately relays the patient's condition and the treatment currently rendered.

3) Describe a patient problem in a manner that appropriately relays the need for further intervention.

4) Discuss initial impression and possible etiologies with progression to probable differential diagnoses.

ACUTE ABDOMINAL PAIN/GI BLEEDING

A The participant will be able to apply critical thinking skills to integrate pathophysiology with assessment and history findings to determine actual and potential patient problems.

KEYS *During a case scenario with an interactive patient, the participant will be able to:*

1) Perform an appropriate assessment.

2) Evaluate for potential risk factors.

3) Evaluate for organ dysfunction.

4) Evaluate for systemic causes.

5) Conduct an appropriate history.

6) Relate medication history to patient problems.

7) Apply pathophysiology to assessment findings.

B Given a scenario or case study, the participant will use problem-solving strategies to determine management alternatives.

KEYS *During a case scenario with an interactive patient, the participant will be able to:*

1) Assess the scene and take appropriate steps for scene management.

2) Initiate immediate management for life-threatening conditions.

3) Differentiate between the different pathophysiological causes of abdominal pain.

4) Differentiate between abdominal organ causes of abdominal pain and referred pain to the abdomen.

5) Differentiate between GI causes of bleeding and other causes.

6) Develop management alternatives for probable differential diagnoses to include as needed: airway management, respiratory and/or ventilatory support, fluid therapy, pharmacological support, and transportation to an appropriate facility.

C The participant will be able to communicate pertinent patient findings and management to medical direction for further orders and to the receiving facility.

KEYS *During a case scenario with an interactive patient, the participant will be able to:*

1) Verbally transmit patient information in an organized manner.

2) Describe a patient problem in a manner that appropriately relays the patient's condition and the treatment currently rendered.

3) Describe a patient problem in a manner that appropriately relays the need for further intervention .

4) Discuss initial impression and possible etiologies with progression to probable differential diagnoses.

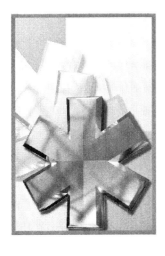

II. ADVANCED MEDICAL LIFE SUPPORT PROVIDER COURSE SLIDE NOTES

The following slides have been identified for use when conducting an NAEMT AMLS course. Each NAEMT AMLS lecture has identified slides that will fulfill the objectives for that lecture. The slide order should not be altered in any way without permission from NAEMT.

CHAPTER 1: ASSESSMENT OF THE MEDICAL PATIENT

SLIDE NO.   **SLIDE TITLE/NOTES**

Slide 1-1   **NAEMT**
The AMLS Program is sponsored by NAEMT. It is endorsed by NAEMSP.

Slide 1-2   **AMLS**
AMLS is an interactive, case-based continuing education course designed to enhance and develop knowledge and skills for the healthcare professional who encounters patients with a variety of medical emergencies.

Slide 1-3   **Provider Course Objectives**
AMLS uses a systematic approach to assessment. This approach allows for a thorough, rapid identification and management of potential life threats.
  ▶ The approach begins with an initial impression and progresses to identifying a differential field diagnosis.
  ▶ Initial management is initiated after the initial assessment and is modified based on information obtained from the focused history and focused physical exam.

Slide 1-4   **Provider Course Objectives**
Review objectives briefly.

Slide 1-5   **Components of AMLS**
  ▶ Interactive, cased-based lectures combined with hands-on teaching stations assist participants with real-time application of the AMLS concepts and skills.
  ▶ Successful completion of the program includes competency in written and scenario-based evaluation stations.

▶ Evaluation stations include: Dyspnea, Chest Pain, Altered Mental Status, and Abdominal Pain/GI Bleeding.

Slide 1-6   **Advanced Medical Life Support**
▶ The AMLS assessment encompasses early recognition and management of life threats.
▶ As information is gathered through history and a physical exam the underlying cause of the event is revealed.

Slide 1-7   **The Assessment of the Medical Patient**
Introduction slide

Slide 1-8   **Introduction**
Review.

Slide 1-9   **Introduction**
▶ Emphasize progression from possibilities to probabilities.

Slide 1-10   **Assessment**
▶ Emphasize the need for dynamic approach and the limited time frame some medical patients have.

Slide 1-11   **Assessment**
▶ Evaluate signs and symptoms to determine life threats. Use your experience and knowledge, scene size-up, and initial impression to determine management priorities.

Slide 1-12   **Assessment**
▶ Your skills in assessment of the medical patient will depend on your ability to collect and rapidly sort information and to make decisions on diagnoses, priorities, and treatment.

Slide 1-13   **The Scene Size-up/BSI**
▶ BSI considerations are infectious disease, tears, amniotic fluid, oozing lesions, urine, saliva, vomit, feces, TB, and MRSA (methicillin-resistant Staphylococcus aureus).
▶ Safety concerns are focused on fumes, hazards, traffic.
▶ Never separate yourself from your partner or radio/cell phone. Realize your limitations.
▶ Signs for a medical patient can be more subtle than a trauma patient.
▶ Don't rule out that a medical patient also may have experienced trauma.

Slide 1-14   **What Is the Scene Telling You?**
▶ Noises may range from domestic disputes to adventitious lung sounds. Odors encompass incontinence, fruity-breath, musty breath, toxic fumes, alcohol abuse, decubitus ulcers, infection.
▶ The chief complaint may not match the signs and symptoms and may reflect altered mental status.
▶ Consider age-, gender-, and race-specific issues: sickle cell anemia, hemophilia, ectopic pregnancy.

Slide 1-15   **Components of Assessment**
▶ Scene size-up/BSI, the initial assessment components of the ABCs, and perfusion are assessment-based approaches.

▶ Initial management begins at this time. The focused history and physical exam along with the detailed physical exam result in a diagnostic-based approach to assessment.
— This "rule in/rule out" of possibilities leads to probabilities and a differential field diagnosis.
— This aspect of assessment modifies the initial management and may include medication administration.
— At this point the underlying etiologies for the differential diagnosis are investigated and identified.

Slide 1-16   **Components of Assessment**
▶ The focused history and physical exam along with the detailed physical exam result in a diagnostic-based approach to assessment.
— This "rule in/rule out" of possibilities leads to probabilities and a differential field diagnosis.
— This aspect of assessment modifies the initial management and may include medication administration.
— At this point the underlying etiologies for the differential diagnosis are investigated and identified.

Slide 1-17   **Focused History**
▶ Assessment of OPQRST and SAMPLE allow for progression from possibilities to probabilities and differential field diagnosis.

Slide 1-18   **Case Study 1**
▶ Concerns are:
— Access in and out from the third floor
— Elderly patient
— The potential for multiple disease processes
— Environmental emergencies
— Toxic fumes
— Additional resources to move patient
— Dependency on assistive devices

Slide 1-19   **Look for the Clues!**
▶ Oxygen equipment is used for cancer, COPD, asthma, cystic fibrosis, chronic lung diseases.
▶ Multiple medication containers can indicate drug toxicity, noncompliance.
▶ Environmental conditions include cleanliness, hydration, nutrition, infection, and poisoning.

Slide 1-20   **Case Study 1**
Ask: *Based on what you see so far, what are your concerns?*
— Female patient appears sick and anxious.
— Possibilities: exacerbation of asthma, CHF, heat-related emergency, hard of hearing/deafness, medication noncompliance or toxicity.
— Lack of hearing can impair communication.

Slide 1-21 **Case Study 1**

▶ Your professional attitude and empathy help develop good communication between you and the patient.

▶ Building good rapport early in the assessment can allow for more trust and the patient sharing historical data.

▶ Utilizing a pleasant tone of voice, touching with permission, and addressing adult patients by their given name can improve rapport and communication.

▶ Paraphrase and restate what the patient tells you to indicate you are listening and understanding.

Slide 1-22 **Case Study 1**

▶ Assessment process for a medical patient begins with the initial assessment, focused history, and physical exam. A trauma patient may require a rapid physical exam prior to obtaining a history.

▶ Life-threat identification and management are determined after the initial assessment components of airway, breathing, circulation/perfusion.

▶ This patient has a potential life threat and is potentially unstable.

Slide 1-23 **Case Study 1**

▶ An altered LOC or compromised airway requires immediate intervention.

▶ Irregular breathing patterns such as Kussmaul's are related to DKA; Cheyne-Stokes are related to CNS dysfunction.

▶ Body positioning (prone, tripod, fetal, flexion [decorticate], extension [decerebrate]) can indicate severity, CVA, increased ICP, seizure, and brain tumor.

▶ Multiple medication containers can indicate drug toxicity, noncompliance.

▶ Environmental concerns include: improperly clothed for temperature, exertion in hot weather, not heating or cooling environment appropriately.

Slide 1-24 **Key Indications of Instability—Airway**

▶ Snoring may indicate tongue is the obstruction; gurgling indicates fluid in upper airway; stridor indicates partial upper airway obstruction; rales indicates fluid; crowing and hoarseness indicate obstruction. Evaluate for vomitus, secretions, blood, edema, or anaphylaxis.

▶ Management may include: manual maneuvers, oral or nasal airways, Combitube, PtL, LMA, or intubation.

Slide 1-25 **Key Indications of Instability—Breathing**

▶ Poor tidal volume decreases alveolar ventilation and leads to poor gas exchange sooner than a slower rate. Retractions of the intercostal spaces, suprasternal notch, supraclavicular spaces, and subcostal area, and asymmetric chest wall movement are indications of instability.

▶ Management includes: oxygen therapy, PPV, and decompression of tension pneumothorax.

Slide 1-26   **Key Indications of Instability—Abnormal Respiratory Patterns**

▶ Kussmaul's indicates signs of acidosis and attempt to compensate for elimination of CO_2; seen in DKA and toxic ingestion.

▶ Biot's and central neurogenic hyperventilation are related to brain injury secondary to stroke, hepatic failure, electrolyte imbalance, and intracranial infection.

▶ Cheyne-Stokes crescendo/decrescendo with apnea indicate CNS dysfunction and brain injury.

Slide 1-27   **Key Indications of Instability—Circulation**

▶ Assess central and peripheral pulses. Weak peripheral pulses indicate hypotension and cardiac dysfunction. Tachycardia/bradycardia may result in decreased cardiac output and decreased perfusion.

▶ Temperature: hot indicates fever, heat emergencies. Cold indicates shock, cold emergencies, and hypothermia.

▶ Bleeds can result from esophageal varices, vaginal and gastrointestinal disorders, past surgery, epistaxis with hypertension. Occult bleeds in elderly may be so minimal they go unnoticed by patient.

▶ Management may include: IV therapy, control of body temperature, Trendelenberg, medication administration such as dopamine.

Slide 1-28   **Altered Mental Status—Pulse Rates**

▶ Irregularity is a clue to dysrhythmias that involve decreased cardiac output and decreased cerebral perfusion. Both cause decreased cardiac output from decreased ventricular filling time. Dysrhythmias can be caused by hypoxia, toxic ingestion, electrolyte disturbances.

▶ Pulse strength is a clue to volume and hydration status.

Slide 1-29   **Key Indications of Instability—CNS**

▶ Two indicators of physiological instability are no spontaneous eye opening and no spontaneous movement to painful stimuli.

▶ Evaluate speech patterns for usage of few words before gasping for breaths which indicate severity. Determine awakeness versus awareness.

▶ Unresponsiveness is always a red flag. Observe for posturing associated with increasing intracranial pressure.

Slide 1-30   **Focused History—Mental Status Assessment**

▶ GCS is essential for medical and trauma patients. Provides a uniform system for determining the patients level of consciousness—more discriminating than AVPU. Also has prognostic value.

▶ AVPU evaluates cognition and orientation.

▶ A GCS less than 8 indicates coma and the need to protect the airway using endotracheal intubation.

▶ GCS of 7–8 has 94% positive outcome.

▶ GCS of 3–4 has 10% positive outcome.

Slide 1-31 **Signs of Advanced Brain Injury**
▶ Flexion of upper extremities—stroke, subdural hematoma, encephalitis, meningitis.
▶ Assess for history of previous head injury or recent fall.

Slide 1-32 **Case Study 1**
▶ AVPU—Stimuli to determine awareness and awakeness
▶ Harriet is also able to correctly state where she is and the time of day.

Slide 1-33 **Case Study 1**
▶ She is unstable or potentially unstable. Respiratory system is initial concern. Chief complaint is difficulty breathing.
▶ Her respiratory distress may be a symptom of underlying environmental emergency or hydration status.

Slide 1-34 **Case Study 1**
▶ Yes, but need to investigate and rule out obstruction and edema.

Slide 1-35 **Case Study 1: Breathing**
▶ Lung sounds that indicate compromise: wheeze; bronchoconstriction related to acute asthma, anaphylaxis; crackles/rales related to fluid in alveoli related to pneumonia, pulmonary edema
▶ Rhonchi are coarse sounds indicating mucus trapped in bronchi related to emphysema, pneumonia, chronic bronchitis.

Slide 1-36 **Case Study 1: Breathing**
▶ Breathing is not adequate. Provide initial oxygen therapy of 15 lpm with NRM and monitor improvement.
▶ If patient deteriorates consider PPV and intubation.
▶ Patient is unstable and should be high transport priority.

Slide 1-37 **Assess Breathing—Potential Respiratory Failure**
▶ Bradypneic related to rate, hypopneic related to depth. PPV and intubation are required for deterioration to respiratory failure. Respiratory failure may result from angioedema, laryngospasm. Signs and symptoms of agitation related to hypoxia must be evaluated for respiratory failure. Treatment requires BVM and RSI.
▶ This patient is in respiratory distress, but is not showing signs of failure at this time.

Slide 1-38 **Circulation and Perfusion Assessment**
▶ Patient remains unstable. Answers to causes on next slide.
▶ Answers may include hypoxia, heat emergency, pneumonia, sepsis, cardiac condition, hypovolemia.

Slide 1-39 **Circulation and Perfusion Assessment**
▶ Review list and verify for which the patient should be evaluated.

Slide 1-40 **Assess the Circulation**
▶ The patient has a radial pulse, so her pressure is at least 80 systolic.

Slide 1-41 **Case Study 1**
▶ Patient is compensating at this time.

Slide 1-42 **Perfusion Assessment—Skin**
▶ Discuss which of these conditions is likely with this patient.

Slide 1-43 **Perfusion Assessment—Capillary Refill**
▶ Since Harriet is older, her perfusion could be compromised by vascular disease and may not be reliable.

Slide 1-44 **Mentation Assessment**
▶ Harriet is alert to verbal stimulus with appropriate verbal response and is not demonstrating cognitive impairment at this time.
— Cognitive impairment is a potential indicator of intracranial pathology (e.g., intracranial bleeds, CVA, infection, seizure, hypoxia, hypertension, and environmental causes such as heat stroke, thiamine deficiency, hypothermia).
— Glasgow Coma Scale—for all patients; not just trauma.
▪ Key components: Eye Opening, Best Motor Response, Best Verbal Response
▪ Lowest score 3, highest 15

Slide 1-45 **Assessing Priorities**
▶ Aggressive management and immediate transport to the appropriate facility are determined at this point in the assessment.
▶ The patient has a serious compromise of her respiratory system and should be transported.
▶ Constant evaluation should be continued and treatment adjusted accordingly.

Slide 1-46 **Establishing Patient Priorities**
▶ Review the list and identify any priorities for transport.

Slide 1-47 **Case Study 1**
▶ Initial impression: respiratory distress with risk for respiratory failure
▶ Differential field diagnosis: exacerbation of chronic asthma, emphysema, chronic bronchitis, or pulmonary edema; heat emergency; sepsis; CHF

Slide 1-48 **Initial Management Considerations**
Review and discuss list.

Slide 1-49 **Focused History/Physical Exam**
▶ The order in which they are performed is determined by the patient's mental status.

Slide 1-50 **Focused History**
▶ As you question the patient, consider the information you can gather from various types of questions.

	SLIDE NO.	SLIDE TITLE/NOTES

Slide 1-51 **Focused History—OPQRST**
- As questions are asked, discuss which diagnoses are being confirmed or rejected as additional information is gathered.

Slide 1-52 **Focused History—OPQRST**
- Positions of comfort indicate severity:
  — Sitting bolt upright
  — Lateral recumbent
  — Fetal position
  — Guarding
- Discuss the implications of patient positioning and patient severity.

Slide 1-53 **Focused History—OPQRST**
- The quality is determined by the patient's perception of difficulty in breathing, pain, etc. Quality encompasses: crushing, tearing, cramping, pressure, dull, sharp, knifelike, ache.
- As questions are asked, discuss which diagnoses are being confirmed or rejected as additional information is gathered.
- Discuss the fact that the patient is elderly, the possibility of ACS (acute coronary syndrome), and the nontraditional presentation.

Slide 1-54 **Focused History—OPQRST**
- An elderly person may feel discomfort and pain everywhere, all the time.
- Have the elderly patient point to the area of greatest discomfort or pain.
- Referred pain is related to the signs and symptoms of kidney stone, gallbladder, AMI, liver and spleen dysfunction.

Slide 1-55 **Focused History—OPQRST**
Discuss which is more likely given her presentation.

Slide 1-56 **Focused History—OPQRST**
- Since the patient is elderly, is on steroids, and has an inhaler, she may have had this condition for a while. Asking her to compare this episode to previous ones may be useful.
- Slow movements, facial affect, moaning, groans, grimacing, and guarding indicate severity. If the patient is unable to find words to describe pain or discomfort, use description scales with faces.

Slide 1-57 **Focused History—OPQRST**
- Duration refers to length of time the signs and symptoms have been present. Determine if the discomfort or pain is constant or intermittent. Discuss the implications of these findings.

Slide 1-58 **Focused History—Past Medical History**
Review briefly.

Slide 1-59 **Focused History—Past Medical History**
- Discuss the implications of the tightness and her being frightened. This may be a red flag for something serious.

Slide 1-60   **Focused History—SAMPLE**
- ▶ Determine allergies to prescription as well as OTC medications.
- ▶ If appears to be anaphylaxis, check allergy to stings, bites, and foods.

Slide 1-61   **Focused History—SAMPLE**
- ▶ Discuss the implications of prednisone and its ability to mask infections, long-term disease, or severe disease process. Additional questions to consider are:
  - — Have you taken your prescribed medications today? If so, how much?
  - — Have you taken any OTC medications today? If so, how much?
  - — Have you taken any new medications today? If so, how much?
- ▶ There can be multiple medication interactions, toxicity related to dosing and noncompliance.

Slide 1-62   **Focused History—SAMPLE**
- ▶ Discuss her answer and the diagnoses generated so far. hypertension, diabetes, cardiovascular disease, respiratory diseases can be factors.

Slide 1-63   **Focused History—SAMPLE**
- ▶ Review. Discuss a capillary blood sugar evaluation and dehydration/nutrition concerns.

Slide 1-64   **Focused History—SAMPLE**
- ▶ Discuss the onset and review the diagnoses for "rule outs."
- ▶ Investigate for exertion, emotional or physically stressful events.

Slide 1-65   **Case Study 1: History**
- ▶ Asthma or COPD likely; use of prednisone may mask infectious response, so pneumonia should be considered. AMI should be kept as an option.

Slide 1-66   **Focused History**
- ▶ Harriet used to smoke, but no longer does. Heat has limited her activity. Denies other factors.
- ▶ Personal habits are closely related to past medical history and can be helpful in determining chronic versus acute signs and symptoms.

Slide 1-67   **Case Study 1: Focused Physical Exam**
- ▶ Yes, the thorax, abdomen, and distal pulses should be more closely evaluated.
- ▶ Harriet's assessment demonstrates some ankle edema, but essentially negative.
- ▶ The rapid medical assessment is conducted systematically and is related to the chief complaint.
- ▶ Assess for surgical scars, implanted devices, lung sounds, work of breathing, pneumothorax, abdominal distention, rigidity, pulsating masses, and rebound tenderness.

SLIDE NO.	SLIDE TITLE/NOTES

Slide 1-68

Case Study 1: Vital Signs

▶ Yes, Harriet's vital signs confirm instability and poor perfusion.

Slide 1-69

Case Study 1: Differential Field Diagnosis

▶ Acute exacerbation of chronic asthma possibly due to the environment.

▶ An AMI may still be a concern as well.

▶ Yes, the differential diagnosis has changed since it has narrowed in focus from possibilities to probabilities.

▶ Differential field diagnosis is a dynamic mental process that requires input and integration of information discovered from every aspect of the scene size-up, history, and physical exam.

Slide 1-70

Case Study 1: Management

Review and discuss treatment. Entertain other options for discussion such as AMI management.

Slide 1-71

Case Study 1: Management

▶ Albuterol relaxes bronchi and smooth muscle by stimulating beta adrenergic receptors.

▶ Methylprednisolone decreases inflammation and suppresses immune response.

▶ Atrovent inhibits vagal-mediated reflexes by antagonizing acetylcholine and muscarinic receptors and bronchial smooth muscle.

▶ Magnesium sulfate relaxes smooth muscle associated with bronchoconstriction.

Slide 1-72

Case Study 1: Ongoing Assessment

▶ Identifies all non-life-threatening conditions.

▶ Done only if time permits and generally done en route to receiving facility. More comprehensive than the focused physical exam.

▶ Ongoing assessment for stable patients is every 15 minutes, for unstable patients every 5 minutes.

▶ Ongoing assessment involves reassessment of the initial assessment, vital signs, and monitoring patient response to interventions.

Slide 1-73

Summary

Ask for questions and summarize.

CHAPTER 2: AIRWAY MANAGEMENT, VENTILATION, AND OXYGEN THERAPY

SLIDE	SLIDE TITLE/NOTES

Slide 2-1   **Airway Management and Ventilation**
- ▶ Airway is a common topic in healthcare education but still the most commonly mismanaged part of emergency care.
- ▶ Oxygen is the key to human life and its main route into the body is the airway.
- ▶ We will presume that your previous education has familiarized you to basic airway management. We will review:
  — Respiratory Anatomy and Physiology
  — Basic and Advanced Airway Adjuncts
  — Medication-Assisted Intubation
  — Failed Intubation Plans
  — Ventilation Techniques

Slide 2-2   **Assessment of the Airway**
- ▶ Medical assessment begins with scene evaluation, an across-the-room assessment of the patient, and then evaluation of the ABCs.
- ▶ Airway assessment begins with a simple conversation in which the healthcare provider introduces him/herself and asks how the patient is. If the patient converses without difficulty, the airway should be patent.
- ▶ If the patient converses with difficulty or does not speak, a more intensive assessment of airway must be initiated. Look for reasons that may threaten the patient's airway: tongue, teeth, blood, secretions, vomitus, etc. Immediate resuscitation of airway threats must take place prior to assessment of the patient's respiratory status.

Slide 2-3   **Airway Interventions**
- ▶ If airway maneuvers need to be performed, the healthcare provider must use basic airway interventions initially and, if an advanced healthcare provider, the organization of future airway needs are based on scope of practice and the situation (e.g., how far away from the hospital are we?).
- ▶ How difficult might it be to intubate this patient?

Slide 2-4   **Indications for Airway Management**
- ▶ Alteration in mental status:
  — Watch carefully for and provide management of the airway.
  — The most common mistake made in airway management is failure to recognize when a patient who is breathing on their own BUT has altered mental status needs airway adjuncts to PROTECT the airway.
- ▶ Hypoxia:
  — The patient in respiratory distress who may be in respiratory failure progresses easily into arrest.
  — Aggressive ventilatory management with airway adjuncts may be needed.

▶ Medical emergency:
— Anticipate that in some medical conditions the patient may need airway management. Be prepared.
— Angioedema and infections are some examples.

Slide 2-5   **Review of Basic Airway Techniques**
▶ Review the basic airway maneuvers as shown with indications, contraindications, and techniques.

Slide 2-6   **Advanced/Alternative Airway Devices**
▶ These advanced airways do not require direct visualization. This is an introductory slide for the next three slides.

Slide 2-7   **Pharyngotracheal Lumen (PtL) Airway**
▶ Dual-lumen (longer tube within a shorter tube) with a stylet and a large oropharyngeal cuff, blindly inserted. Describe the use of this device. Reinforce that attaching the strap around patient's head is essential in proper positioning of this device.
▶ Device is contraindicated in caustic ingestion and known esophageal disease.

Slide 2-8   **Esophageal Tracheal Combitube Airway**
▶ Diagram showing the Combitube in both the esophageal and tracheal positions.
▶ Similar to the PtL but the dual-lumen tubes are side-by-side with a cuff on each tube.
▶ Describe the use of this device. The Combitube has the same indications and contraindications as the PtL. Emphasize that it requires the same skills and practice as the PtL.

Slide 2-9   **Laryngeal Mask Airway (LMA) Unique (disposable)**
▶ The LMA is a blindly-inserted, advanced airway device that is relatively new on the market. It can be used in various sizes in all age groups with very few contraindications to its use. (NOTE: Requires skill and practice to use the device).
▶ LMA-Unique is used as a bridging device to endotracheal intubation in the emergency setting. It does not protect against aspiration of gastric contents, although, when used, provides better bag-valve ventilation tidal volumes with no increased risk of aspiration over using the BVM by itself.

Slide 2-10   **Insertion Technique for the LMA**
▶ The preferred technique for insertion is described on this slide.
▶ A thorough description of this technique is provided on the LMA of North America web site (www.lmana.com).

Slide 2-11   **Advanced Airway Techniques**
Each technique will be discussed on the following slides.

Slide 2-12   **Quality Assurance for Endotracheal Intubation**
▶ Advanced healthcare providers who are credentialed to provide endotracheal intubation should assure themselves enough practice in this technique in order to become proficient, especially if considering using medications to enhance patient compliance.

▶ In order to maintain proficiency in this skill, performing 6–12 intubations per year (adult) is a minimum recommendation from the American Heart Association and the Society for Anesthesiology.

Slide 2-13   LMA-Fastrach

▶ The LMA-Fastrach is a specially designed LMA that allows an 8.0 mm ETT to be inserted without visualization. Insertion technique is similar to the LMA-Unique but the stainless steel adaptor guides blind ETT insertion.

▶ Again, this device requires skill and practice—preferably in the operating room under the guidance of an anesthesiologist.

Slide 2-14   Nasotracheal Intubation

▶ Review the pros and cons.

▶ Use of this technique is appropriate as an alternative to orotracheal intubation when the patient:
  — Cannot be placed into a supine position
  — Is lethargic but not unconscious
  — Has difficulties with swelling or secretions in the oropharynx (inhibits visualization)
  — Has a clenched jaw

▶ This technique, however, does require skill and practice. Success rate is fairly low and soft-tissue injury usually occurs.

▶ Delayed consequences of nasotracheal intubation:
  — Small tubes (remember the smaller the diameter of the tube, the more airway compromise)
  — Complication rates higher

Slide 2-15   Digital and Lighted-Stylet Intubation

▶ Both techniques are essentially "blind" in that direct visualization is not performed.

▶ Lighted stylet:
  — ET tube with lighted stylet advanced into larynx
  — Neck must be shielded from light source.
  — Less risk to the healthcare provider than digital

▶ Digital technique:
  — Historically, the first way we intubated.
  — Patient MUST be without any gag reflex.
  — Epiglottis is palpated as 2 to 3 fingers are inserted into lower oropharynx (walk down the tongue).
  — ETT (with stylet shaped into hockey stick or L) inserted behind fingers—2nd finger traps progressing ETT and guides it above identified epiglottis. Stop at intervals and remove portions of inserted stylet as you advance ETT distally.

Slide 2-16   Lighted-Stylet Intubation

▶ A review of the steps. Note the placement of the fingers and the need to adapt this skill for digital intubation without stylet.

	SLIDE NO.	SLIDE TITLE/NOTES

Slide 2-17   **Alternative Airways: Surgical**
▶ This is an introductory slide. These techniques are described in subsequent slides.
▶ Indications for surgical airway:
 — ETT cannot be achieved
 — Anatomic deformities (previous head/neck surgery)
 — Direct obstruction of upper airway (edema or FBAO)

NOTE: Discussing these techniques does not authorize their use. Many regions do not allow EMS to provide these techniques.

Slide 2-18   **Surgical Airways: Percutaneous Transtracheal Jet Ventilation**
▶ High-pressure oxygen driven into the tracheobronchial tree as a TEMPORARY or bridge to a more definitive airway
 — The problem is CO_2 retention.
 — Limit of 30–45 minutes for this ventilation technique
 — Need at least 50 psi to deliver the oxygen and ventilate
 — Many modifications used to provide tubing with ventilation ports (including manufactured products)
 — Complications include bleeding and hematoma formation; esophageal entrance with contamination of the mediastinum; infection; further airway compromise; damage to the thyroid gland; and subcutaneous emphysema

Slide 2-19   **Surgical Airways: Retrograde Intubation**
The same anatomic location must be identified with this procedure as with percutaneous needle insufflation.
▶ In this technique, the needle is angled towards the head.
▶ A 24-inch+ J-wire is required and is inserted through properly inserted needle until it can be visualized in the patient's mouth. Grasp wire with clamp and pull up and out of mouth, but DO NOT pull end of wire completely out of the needle.
▶ Insert guide wire through eye of distal ETT and pull ETT through mouth and into position where resistance is met near glottis.
▶ As guide wire is removed, apply gentle downward pressure on distal tip of positioned ETT to guide it into vocal cords. Inflate cuff of ETT and confirm placement.
▶ Retrograde intubation requires a great deal of dexterity, skill, and time.

Slide 2-20   **Surgical Cricothyrotomy**
NOTE: This may be a procedure that is not allowed in your EMS region. The healthcare provider should consider BVM ventilation until the patient can be delivered to the resources necessary to provide this advanced airway technique in a more controlled environment.
▶ Steps to surgical cricothyrotomy:
 — Insert ETT into surgical incision. ETT should be sized 1 mm less than would normally be inserted orotracheally.

— Must maintain patency of surgical incision with either a finger, clamp, etc. while ETT inserted. You may use commercially available devices, according to directions.

— Complications include hemorrhage, infection, etc.

Slide 2-21   **Assessment of Ventilation**

▶ Once the patient's airway is open, assess the patient's minute volume. Assess a general rate and work of breathing:

— Quiet tachypnea (fast but not labored) is a sign of sympathetic nervous stimulation, such as shock.

— Labored breathing may be an indication of many major life-threatening illnesses.

▶ Once a sense of the patient's rate and work of breathing is assessed, assess the patient's tidal volume—is it adequate? Auscultation of breath sounds in the apices helps determine that air is moving in the lower airways and the patient is taking deep enough breaths for adequate tidal volume.

▶ For those patients presenting with extremes in respiratory rates (bradypnea, tachypnea) or with poor tidal volume, assisted ventilation may need to be provided.

▶ As you are assessing the patient in the initial assessment—use of monitoring devices is not advisable. Once the focused exam is initiated, cardiac and respiratory monitoring devices can be used to help gather data about the patient's overall status. These devices, by themselves, are not to be used to determine whether a patient needs to have assisted ventilation or oxygen therapy.

Slide 2-22   **Capnography**

▶ In addition to cardiac monitoring and pulse oximetry, capnography may be a monitoring tool in the assessment of the patient's respiratory status.

▶ Colormetric devices vs. capnography with waveform technology must be evaluated by your healthcare service for the type that is appropriate for your environment. No matter which type of carbon dioxide detection technology is chosen, it is important that all types be understood fully by healthcare providers.

Slide 2-23   **Review of Ventilation Techniques**

▶ Techniques listed on the slide:

— BVM with 2–3 persons AND cricoid pressure (discussed in next 2 slides). Mimic a natural inspiratory and expiratory cycle when ventilating the patient via BVM.

— CPAP (continuous positive airway pressure) is positive pressure applied throughout the respiratory cycle to the spontaneously breathing patient with reliable ventilatory drive and adequate tidal volume. This device enhances oxygenation to the patient, similar to PEEP.

▪ This type of non-invasive pressure support ventilation (NIPSV) may also be known as BiPAP (bilevel positive airway pressure).

— Flow-restricted, oxygen-powered devices and techniques should again mimic a natural inspiratory/expiratory cycle and there is no indication of lung compliance with this device.

— Pocket mask with supplemental oxygen and positive pressure may actually provide better tidal volume and less barotrauma than other devices.

— One-person BVM is very difficult and may be the least effective method.

NOTE: Discuss these methods but reinforce the fact that all techniques should not cause high-pressure, forceful inspiratory phases with no chance at exhalation (which should be at least at a 1:2 ratio). **All positive pressure ventilation without a protected airway will cause gastric insufflation unless precautions are taken.**

Slide 2-24   **Basic Ventilation Techniques**

▶ Pocket mask (as discussed on previous slide) usually provides better tidal volume than use of bag-valve mask (BVM), especially if used by only one rescuer. Adding supplemental oxygen to the pocket-mask device adds to this basic ventilation tool for a single rescuer.

▶ In bag-valve-mask ventilation, ideally one rescuer provides a mask seal on the patient's face (EC clamp technique) and another rescuer provides positive pressure ventilation at a rate of 12/minute for the adult. Adding supplemental oxygen and oxygen reservoir devices enhance oxygenation to the patient while providing ventilation.

▶ Cricoid pressure should be provided during all positive pressure ventilations in order to prevent passive regurgitation.

Slide 2-25   **Recap**

▶ This slide reinforces the "slow and low" ventilation procedures advocated for BVM.

▶ This slide mentions hyperventilation techniques that may be used for the patient exhibiting signs of cerebral herniation in the late stages of increased intracranial pressure processes.

▶ Note that the rate of ventilation only increases to 15–20 per minute for this treatment and should be guided by end-tidal CO_2 monitoring whenever available since there is a very narrow range of CO_2 allowed for this practice.

Slide 2-26   **Cricoid Pressure/Sellick's Maneuver**

▶ Landmarks of the anatomy

▶ Use the thyroid cartilage as a landmark to find the cricoid— NOT as a location for pressure.

▶ The dominant thumb and forefinger should be used on the lateral borders of the cricoid ring.

Slide 2-27   **Cricoid Pressure Effects**

▸ Pressure is applied posteriorly for this maneuver, preventing higher pressures of air from ventilation techniques entering the esophagus, thus preventing regurgitation and aspiration of gastric contents. This technique, in conjunction with all positive pressure techniques, *requires an effective mask seal.*

▸ An adaptation of this maneuver may be used to assist those attempting to view the vocal cords during endotracheal intubation and should not be released until the cuff is inflated on the endotracheal tube.

Slide 2-28   **Continuous Positive Airway Pressure (CPAP)**

▸ Continuous positive airway pressure is positive pressure applied throughout the entire respiratory cycle via inspiratory and expiratory positive pressure.

▸ The patient must be spontaneously breathing with reliable ventilatory drive and adequate tidal volume.

▸ Indications:
  — Ventilation support for those difficult to oxygenate because of conditions that reduce the functional residual capacity, such as congestive heart failure with pulmonary edema, atelectasis, or secretion retention
  — Patients with airway edema or obstructive disease who need to maintain adequate ventilation
  — Used in the hospital as a means of weaning patients from pressure support ventilators

▸ Non-invasive pressure support ventilation (NIPSV), also known as bilevel positive airway pressure (BiPAP) ventilation, is a noninvasive mode of ventilation in which there is both a set level of inspiratory and expiratory positive airway pressure. This may be applied through a nose mask.

Slide 2-29   **Introduction to RSI**

Slide 2-30   **Medication-Assisted Intubation (RSI) Procedures**

▸ Staged induction intubation (RSI) (This is not a rapid procedure!)

▸ Pose these two questions and provide support for pertinent answers prior to moving on.

Ask: *What procedures need to be completed in order to assure that this intubation will be successful?*

Ask: *What QA procedures should be in place in your system in order to prepare you for this procedure?*
  — Performer knows limitations; has proven competency to Medical Director.
  — Assesses the patient adequately for anatomic, physiologic contraindications to this technique.
  — Has several backup plans in case the intubation cannot be performed once paralysis has been induced.

Slide 2-31 — The Steps to Successful RSI

▶ **P**reparation: assessment, fall-back plans, monitors, IVs (2 is best), supplies, equipment, position
▶ **P**re-Oxygenation: (Provides an oxygen reservoir within the lungs. Washes out nitrogen, allowing for more apnea time). 90–100% oxygen for at least 5 minutes. Try NOT to use BVM unless patient requires ventilation support prior to intubation (helps prevent aspiration).
▶ **P**re-Treatment: With drugs used to minimize intubation side-effects:
— **L**idocaine: for reactive airway disease and elevated ICP
— **O**pioid: to blunt sympathetic response
— **A**tropine: for children and relative bradycardia
— **D**efasciculation of Succinylcholine: for elevated ICP, high gastric pressures, eye injuries
▶ **P**aralysis with Induction: Sedative and paralytic—both short-acting, short half-life drugs
▶ **P**rotection and Positioning: Sellick's maneuver, then position head/neck for intubation
▶ **P**lacement and Proof: Intubate, inflate the cuff, then use two means of ETT confirmation.
▶ **P**ost-Intubation Management: Secure ETT, ventilate, chest X ray, end-tidal CO_2 capnography, and monitor vital signs; long-term sedation and paralysis.

Slide 2-32 — Pre-RSI Anatomic Assessment

▶ 3-3-2 Rule
— Anatomic assessment of the patient in an attempt to answer the question: Can I intubate this patient?
— Geometry of oral intubation: The first 3 of the 3-3-2 rule is three fingers between the teeth (can it open adequately?); the second 3 is measurement of the space from the mentum to the hyoid bone (diagram in previous slide) and identifies access to the airway. The 2 in the 3-3-2 rule requires two fingers be placed between the thyroid notch and the floor of the mandible. This identifies that the larynx is sufficiently low within the neck to permit oral access.

Slide 2-33 — Pre-RSI Assessment

▶ Prior to giving medications . . .

Ask: *Can I intubate this patient?*
— An anatomic assessment should be performed (pre-RSI procedure).

Slide 2-34 — Mallampati Assessment, Pre-RSI

▶ This identifies the amount of space available within the mouth for the insertion of both the laryngoscope and an ETT.
▶ The ideal patient position for this exam is a High Fowler's position with head in sniffing position and the patient sticking out their tongue.
▶ If the patient must be supine, use a tongue blade to mimic the tongue depression.

Slide 2-35   Pre-RSI Procedures
- ▶ Another mnemonic, LEMON, helps in assuring success in RSI.
- ▶ NOTE: Mallampati assessment described on previous slide.
- ▶ Neck mobility: Attempt to take head/neck through range of motion (medical patient only), especially in the elderly. Patient places chin to chest, looks at the floor, then the ceiling.

Slide 2-36   Pre-Treatment Drugs for RSI: LOAD
- ▶ Review of drugs that may be given prior to sedation and paralysis (induction).

Slide 2-37   General Procedures for RSI
- ▶ Review the steps in medication-assisted intubation (RSI).
- ▶ Reinforce the length of time this procedures takes. ***This is not a rapid procedure!***

Slide 2-38   SOAP ME Format—RSI Procedure
- ▶ Another mnemonic for remembering the steps in RSI: SOAP ME as described on the slide.
- ▶ Reinforce that oxygen is added early so that nitrogen can be washed out.

Slide 2-39   Failed Intubation Protocols
- ▶ 99–100% of emergency department RSI procedures are successful because of the resources available as backup plans.
- ▶ The AHA cites a 50% failure rate amongst EMS systems with a low patient volume.
- ▶ Somewhere in between those two statistics for success rates in endotracheal intubation, the healthcare provider sees the need for backup plans if the intubation is not successful.

  Ask: *Besides going "back to the basics," what are some procedures we can perform if the endotracheal tube is not properly inserted after giving sedatives and paralytics in a staged intubation attempt?*
- ▶ Support discussion:
  - — LMA, Combitube, PtL (remind them of the short-acting paralytic and use of esophageal tubes)
  - — A second rescuer who is competent at intubating
  - — Digital intubation while patient is still paralyzed
  - — Cricothyrotomy (last resort)

  Ask: *How long will the effects last for most sedatives/paralytics given in the initial induction?*

  NOTE: Be patient here, allow for quick reference checks and book review with discussion.

Slide 2-40   Failed Intubation Procedures
Recap—provides some of the answers to first question on slide 2-39.

Slide 2-41   **Paralytic Duration of Action**
Recap—provides major answers to second question on slide 2-39.

Slide 2-42   **Case Study 1: The Unconscious Female**
▶ Have participants read the case on their own. Provide a synopsis of the information as it is displayed.

Ask: *What does this scene tell you?*
▶ Scene size-up:
    — Entrance and exit available for your team?
    — Critical vs. non-critical situation?
    — Interpersonal dynamics?
▶ Stress that this patient is demonstrating "at risk" behavior, which places her at greater risk for communicable diseases.

NOTE: Do not move to the next slide until the answers are discussed.

Slide 2-43   **Case Study 1: Initial Assessment**
▶ General impression with ABCD. Have a participant read the information as you provide a synopsis.

Ask: *What would your initial treatment be?*
▶ Allow participants to discuss/provide potential answers.
    — Provide quick and simple airway positioning.
    — Suction.
    — Use pocket mask (with eventual oxygen) or BVM (with eventual oxygen) to immediately provide positive pressure ventilation. This will also help resuscitate the shock patient in bradycardia.
▶ Ask the related question below and discuss before moving on to the next slide.

Ask: *Should you treat the unstable patient or gather history?*
    — The unstable patient must have initial (basic) resuscitation prior to gathering history. (Review from Assessment/ Management lecture.)

Slide 2-44   **Case Study 1**
Provides an outline of the answers to the previous slide's questions. Recap the initial assessment.

Slide 2-45   **Additional Information**
Transition slide from the initial assessment to the SAMPLE history

Slide 2-46   **Case Study 1**
▶ Have participants read as you provide synopsis of information—reinforcing SAMPLE and OPQRST format.

Ask: *What does this information tell you?*
    — Unconsciousness is the chief complaint, therefore many of the history questions are not applicable.
▶ Read and discuss prior to asking next question.
    — Initial field impression
    — Differential impressions

Ask: *What part of the assessment should you do now?*
— Focused physical exam
— Possibly some OPQRST questions

Slide 2-47 **Field Impression**
Recap—provides an outline of the answers regarding the
SAMPLE and OPQRST assessments.

Slide 2-48 **Focused Physical Exam**
▶ Have participants read as you provide synopsis of information—reinforcing the Focused Physical Exam and forming
a field impression with differential diagnosis.

Ask: *What is your field impression? What other differential
diagnoses could this be?*
▶ Discuss possible differential diagnoses.
▶ Have participants provide answers prior to asking next
question.

Ask: *What would your initial treatment be?*
▶ Discuss prior to next slide.

Slide 2-49 **Field Impression**
Recap—answers first question from slide 2-48.

Slide 2-50 **Immediate Plan of Care**
Recap—answers second question from slide 2-48.

Slide 2-51 **Case Study 1**
▶ Have participants read the information, which you may also
summarize.

Ask: *At what rate and depth should you ventilate this patient?*
▶ Discuss potential answers below prior to reading the next
question. Demonstrate while counting so participants realize the "slow and low" ventilations that should be delivered.
— Rate of 12–15/minute with inspiratory cycle over 1.5 to
2 seconds
— The ratio of inspiratory to expiratory time should be 1:2
(meaning that the inspiration should last 1.5 to 2.0 seconds and exhalation should occur over 3-4 seconds)

Ask: *What are some basic airway adjuncts that could be used
for this patient?*
— Oropharyngeal airway
— Nasopharyngeal airway
— Esophageal tubes (PtL, DualLumen tube)
— Laryngeal airways
— Always have suction available

Slide 2-52 **Case Study 1**
▶ Review with participants.

Ask: *What are some advanced airway adjuncts that could be
used?*
▶ Discuss prior to asking the next question on the slide.

NOTES	SLIDE NO.	SLIDE TITLE/NOTES

Ask: *What are some of the contraindications to using the airway devices you have mentioned?*

▶ Discuss contraindications as participants provide the name of an acceptable advanced airway in this case.

Slide 2-53   **Case Study 1**

▶ Review the information so far: Patient gagged on an oral airway, has GCS of 5, is high risk for aspiration, and also needs to receive positive pressure ventilation.

NOTE: In order to meet the objectives, tell the participants that the decision has been made to intubate.

Ask: *Does this patient need to be sedated prior to intubation?*

NOTE: Discuss first question prior to asking the second question on the slide.

▶ Take some time here. This can be controversial and participants will need guidance.

▶ Final answer depends on local protocols; one could argue that the patient has probably already been sedated.

▶ However, sedation in normal doses does not eliminate the gag reflex. The patient may bite down (reflexively) on the laryngoscope blade due to gag action.

Ask: *Will this patient need to receive a paralytic drug (along with sedation) prior to intubation?*

▶ Review indications for medication-assisted intubation, along with contraindications.

Slide 2-54   **Case Study 1**

▶ To meet objective, first discuss medication-assisted intubation with sedation only.

Ask: *What might you expect with sedation only for side effects/complications?*

— Tight airway due to intact gag reflex

— Side effects from the sedative used (see PDR)

Ask: *What should we do now?*

▶ Allow for guided discussion prior to the next slide.

Slide 2-55   **Options**

Recap procedures used when sedation only does not allow for successful intubation.

Slide 2-56   **Case Study 1**

▶ Review update information with participants.

▶ Review depth of placement procedures for ETT.

Ask: *What cm marking should be at the patient's lip?*

— Generally 3 times the tube size (±1)

Ask: *What confirmation procedures should be used for ETT placement?*

— 3–5 point auscultation

— End-tidal CO_2 detection (colormetric, capnography)

— Esophageal tube check

Slide 2-57   **Intubation Assessment Devices**

Recap of answer to question 2 on slide 2-56.

▶ Esophageal tube check: Creates a suction force at the tracheal (distal) end of the ETT, either by pulling back on a plunger of a syringe or compressing a bulb. It is based on the ability to readily aspirate air from the cartilage-supported trachea by drawing from gas in the lower airways.

— Not reliable in patients younger than 4–5 years of age, who are morbidly obese, or those in late pregnancy.

▶ Exhaled or end-tidal CO_2 monitoring: a colormetric device attached between the positioned ETT and the positive pressure ventilation device.

— Ventilate patient at a normal rate for 6 cycles before assessing the true color of the device.

▪ Yellow indicates CO_2 is being detected—the ETT should be in the trachea.

▪ Tan means that there may be poor blood flow to the lungs.

— Ventilate 6 more times and recheck color; find the cause for poor lung perfusion (PE, Arrest).

▪ If the color remains purple in a patient with a pulse (good perfusion), the ETT is probably in the esophagus. If the patient's lungs are receiving poor or no blood flow, this device may be unreliable.

Slide 2-58   **Case Study 1**

▶ Remind participants of the status of this case. The patient has been successfully intubated and position has been assured via two methods.

▶ Ask and discuss this question before showing and discussing the second question on the slide.

Ask: *What rate and tidal volume should we ventilate this patient?*

— "Slow and low" is advocated. A rate of about 12 per minute with a tidal volume that just barely allows the chest to rise slowly, over 1–2 seconds. Normal lungs are usually set at an inspiratory/expiratory ratio of 1:2.

NOTE: It is sometimes helpful to demonstrate with your hands (mimick holding a BVM) the 1–2 second duration. Inspiratory time at a ratio of 1:2 at a rate of 10–12 per minute.

Ask: *If monitoring patient's CO_2 levels, what measurement is ideal?*

— Continuous capnography measurements (if available) should show a normal level (35–45 mmHg) unless specifically directed by Medical Direction.

Slide 2-59   **Ventilation Considerations**

Recap of answers to questions on previous slide.

NOTE: You may need to explain "herniation syndrome" as it applies to increasing ICP. This procedure for hyperventilation

is protocol driven and specific to finding Cushing's reflex with pupil changes—and is thought of as a resuscitation to prevent herniation of the brain through the foramen magnum. Allowing the CO_2 levels to fall below 35 for an extended period of time dramatically decreases blood flow to the brain.
▶ Provide summary of Case Study 1.

Slide 2-60   **Case Study 2**
Present if time allows.

Slide 2-61   **Case Study 2: Scene Size-up**
▶ Provide a synopsis of this case as participants read it. This is a postcode patient who is being ventilated via ETT.

Slide 2-62   **Case Study 2**
Ask: *What complication could be occurring?*
▶ Discuss answers to this question prior to viewing and discussing the next question on this slide.

Ask: *What complications occur suddenly in the intubated patient?*

Ask: *What actions should be taken to correct this problem?*
▶ As participants offer answers to question 1, go back and ask what they would do to correct it.
▶ Reinforce the need for securing ETT and routine reassessment for depth of placement (cm mark at the lip) as simple head/torso movement can completely dislodge an ETT.

Slide 2-63   **Complication in the Intubated Patient**
▶ This mnemonic, DOPE, is taken from the AHA's PALS course.
   — It is a quick way to remember what can go wrong in an intubated patient.

Slide 2-64   **Case Study 2**
Ask: *What should be done to correct the problem?*

Slide 2-65   **Complications in the Intubated Patient**
▶ Review the sudden and severe complications that may occur in the intubated patient. Review procedures to correct the problem.

Slide 2-66   **Summary**
End of Case Study 2.

Slide 2-67   **References**

CHAPTER 4: HYPOPERFUSION (SHOCK)

SLIDE	SLIDE TITLE/NOTES

Slide 4-1 **Hypoperfusion**
Introduction

Slide 4-2 **Physiological Changes in Response to Shock**
▶ Discuss the physiological changes that occur in response to shock.
▶ As cardiac output drops (for whatever reason), baroreceptors in the arch of the aorta sense the change and stimulate the systemic response:
  — Sympathetic nervous system stimulates the adrenal medullae to secrete catecholamines.
  — Catecholamines secreted and stimulate alpha and beta receptors sites in heart, lungs, blood vessels, and sweat glands to cause:
    ▪ vasoconstriction
    ▪ bronchodilation
    ▪ increased heart rate
    ▪ increased cardiac contraction
▶ As decreased oxygen and glucose supplies to cells continue:
  — Kidneys sense a drop in pressure and release Renin.
  — Renin stimulates the production of Angiotensin I.
  — Angiotensin I is converted to Angiotensin II, which is a powerful vasoconstrictor.
  — Angiotensin II stimulates the production of Aldosterone, which acts on the kidney to conserve water.

Slide 4-3 **Alpha and Beta Receptor Site Activity Within Sympathetic Nervous System**
▶ Review the determinates of BP (CO × PVR) and their relationship to alpha stimulation.
▶ Illustrate to participants the ease of using the CARDIO mnemonic in remembering beta properties.
▶ Relates these activities to the signs and symptoms of shock.

Slide 4-4 **Cell Death in Shock**
▶ Walk participants through the steps in cell death in shock; discuss what happens in each step.
  — Shift from aerobic to anaerobic metabolism
  — Failure of Na-ATP pump with intracellular accumulation of Na
  — Intracellular swelling including cellular mitochondria, resulting in further loss of cellular energy sources
  — Breakdown of lysosomes with cellular destruction and death
▶ Remind participants that a collection of like cells make up tissues, like tissues make up organs, like organs make up systems. As more and more cells die, so do tissues, organs, and then systems.

	SLIDE NO.	SLIDE TITLE/NOTES

Slide 4-5   **Factors in the Severity of Shock**
- ▶ Type of shock: Anaphylactic shock may appear within minutes while septic shock may take days to appear.
- ▶ Age of patient: In younger patients, it takes less to induce shock. In older patients, the compensatory mechanisms may take longer to begin response.
- ▶ Pre-existing disorders: Compensatory mechanism may be malfunctioning or not functioning at all.
- ▶ Speed of onset: The slower the onset, the more time for the patient to compensate.
- ▶ Effects of drugs and other substances: Drugs such as beta blockers, ACE inhibitors, and others may block portions of the compensatory response. Alcohol and other recreation drugs can interfere with the body's normal response to shock, or even result in neurogenic shock.

Slide 4-6   **A Review of the Four Major Types of Shock**
- ▶ It is essential that the organs or systems be reviewed to identify the cause of shock so that the appropriate treatment can be initiated.

Slide 4-7   **Hemorrhagic Shock**
- ▶ Compensated (early) hemorrhagic shock signs and symptoms. You may want to relate these (again) to the pathophysiology of shock discussed earlier in this presentation.

Slide 4-8   **Progressive Hemorrhagic Shock**
- ▶ Compensation mechanisms begin to recede as blood loss continues in hemorrhagic shock—related to these signs and symptoms.

NOTE: The symptoms displayed here should be related to the previously discussed pathophysiology and response in shock.
- ▶ Point out that BP begins to fall in this phase.

NOTE: Classic shock signs should be a review for participants.

Slide 4-9   **Irreversible Hemorrhagic Shock**
- ▶ Irreversible shock signs and symptoms in hemorrhagic shock reflect the circulation of acids, enzymes, microemboli with cell damage and death . . . organ failure.
- ▶ Tell participants they will now compare the signs and symptoms of hemorrhagic shock (previously taught as classic shock) to those of anaphylactic shock.

Slide 4-10   **Comparison of Anaphylactic to Hemorrhagic Shock**
- ▶ State that there are many different agents that can cause an anaphylactic reaction.
- ▶ Route of exposure can be via injection, ingestion, absorption, or inhalation.
- ▶ Anaphylactic shock is a form of distributive shock.
- ▶ Emphasize that it is an exaggerated immune response that along with a distributive shock causes angioedema to the airway.

▶ Mast cells release histamine, SRSA (slow reacting substance of anaphylaxis), heparin, platelet-activating factors, and other chemicals that cause widespread vasodilation and blood vessel leaking (flushed skin with hives, petechia, and itching).

▶ Vessel permeability also causes widespread edema, especially in the mucous membranes (wheezing, stridor, rales).

▶ Smooth muscle contraction in GI tract may result in cramping, vomiting, and diarrhea.

▶ Profound hypotension with dyspnea is a common presentation.

▶ Discuss the onset of signs and severity of reaction.
— Speed of the reaction depends on the degree of sensitivity the patient has previously developed, route of exposure, and the target organ.
— Healthcare provider can anticipate that if time of exposure and onset of symptoms are close together, the overall reaction will be severe.

Slide 4-11   **Hypovolemic Shock vs. Hemorrhagic Shock**

Ask: *What types of medical conditions can present with non-hemorrhagic hypovolemic shock?*
— Nonketotic hyperosmolar coma
— DKA
— Gastrointestinal losses
— Third spacing

▶ Review the physiologic changes of aging and signs of shock.

NOTE: Segue into next slide by stating that there are four categories of shock; let's look at obstructive shock next.

Slide 4-12   **Obstructive Shock**

▶ Describe the pathophysiology behind the inability of the myocardium to adequately fill due to the pressure exerted on it or the blockages preventing the flow of blood—interference with preload and afterload.

▶ Cardiac tamponade causes inadequate filling pressure of the heart.

▶ Pulmonary embolism and tension pneumothorax result in inadequate venous return to the heart.

Slide 4-13   **Pulmonary Embolus**

Ask: *What conditions increase the risk of pulmonary embolism?*
— Obesity
— Recent immobility or recent surgery
— Patient taking oral contraceptives, especially among smokers
— Hereditary coagulation disorders

▶ Pulmonary embolus interferes with preload to the left ventricle.

▶ Chest pain is not always present—if it is, it is usually pleuritic in nature.

▶ Lung sounds are usually clear.

▶ Certain clot showers may create syncope and cardiac arrest, arrhythmias like PVCs, and atrial fibrillation.

▶ Treatment is generally supportive in the prehospital setting.

Slide 4-14 **Cardiac Tamponade**

▶ Point out that tamponade is usually associated with a trauma etiology.

Ask: *What medical conditions can cause a pericardial tamponade?*
— Pericardial effusion (inflammatory, infectious, neoplastic)
— Rare outside of trauma

▶ Pericardial tamponade restricts cardiac filling.

▶ May present with a paradoxical pulse with hypoxia.

▶ Beck's Triad is the classic presentation: narrowed pulse pressure, distended neck veins, and distant heart sounds.

▶ Point out the difficulties inherent in assessing for Beck's Triad in the field.

▶ Point out the major clinical differentiation of diminished breath sounds in tension pneumothorax vs. tamponade.

NOTE: Whether prehospital personnel can perform pericardiocentesis or not, it is important for the provider to identify and report these symptoms and the history that supports the development of this condition.

Slide 4-15 **Tension Pneumothorax**

Ask: *What medical conditions can lead to a tension pneumothorax?*
— COPD—ruptured bleb
— Over-inflation injuries

▶ The most common cause of pneumothorax is a mechanically ventilated patient.

▶ Differentiate between signs and symptoms of a simple pneumothorax, tension pneumothorax, and pericardial tamponade.

▶ Positive pressure ventilation should not be withheld from patients with a tension pneumothorax, but the provider must understand that the condition will worsen.

▶ Definitive treatment is needle decompression.

▶ Review the correct procedure for this critical treatment.

NOTE: Segue to the next slide, which reviews the next type of shock, distributive, which was partially covered in the first case study.

Slide 4-16 **Distributive Shock**

▶ The problem is not a decreased volume or obstructed flow of blood, but rather an extreme vasodilation and increased capillary permeability, causing a relative hypovolemia.

▶ Not enough fluid to fill the larger tank.

Slide 4-17   **Neurogenic Shock**
Ask: *What medical conditions can result in neurogenic shock?*
— Toxins from infections and poisons
— Extreme parasympathetic discharge from an overdose
— Association with traumatic injury to the spinal column or spinal cord

▶ Widespread vasodilation is usually due to loss of sympathetic response. The signs and symptoms differ from "classic" shock because of this pathophysiology. Skin vitals do not fit the picture! Heart rate does not fit the picture!

▶ Pulmonary edema may occur with drug or poison-induced shock along with severe compromise in respirations.

▶ Treatment is aimed at supporting the dilated vessels and administration of an antidote. Follow local protocols for antidote but naloxone, glucagon, diazepam, flumazenil may be considered. If lungs are clear, controlled fluid boluses may be considered until vasopressors may be administered.

Slide 4-18   **Septic Shock**
▶ Result of an overwhelming infection
▶ Release of bacterial or viral toxins that cause vasodilation and increased permeability
▶ Discuss potential causes, such as:
— Respiratory infections
— Decubitus ulcers
— Urinary tract infections

▶ There may be a wide variety of symptoms, depending on the organism, strength of the patient's immune system, inflammatory response, and the involved tissues/organs. First stage is hypermetabolism; last stage is shock.

▶ The very young and very old may not present with fever.

▶ DO NOT confuse the symptoms of dyspnea with changes in lung sounds with CHF.

▶ Multi-system organ dysfunction many times is the result of this type of shock with widespread microemboli.

▶ Treatment is aimed at early antibiotic coverage with vessel support, with first judicious fluid administration, and vasopressor drugs.

NOTE: Segue to the next slide on cardiogenic shock.

Slide 4-19   **Cardiogenic Shock**
Ask: *What are the causes of cardiogenic shock besides an AMI?*
— Valvular insufficiency
— Rhythm disturbances

▶ If caused by an AMI, then at least 40% of the myocardium will be damaged.

NOTES	SLIDE NO.	SLIDE TITLE/NOTES

Slide 4-20 **Cardiogenic Shock vs. Hemorrhagic**
▶ Emphasize the differences between cardiogenic and hypovolemic shock.
— You *must* be able to differentiate the two because the treatment of each can be fatal if employed for the wrong pathophysiological condition.
— Aggressive fluid therapy can be fatal in the presence of cardiogenic shock, and vasopressors can be harmful if inadequate fluid resuscitation is present in hypovolemic shock. Emphasize the findings of orthopnea and PND.
▶ Review the standards in pharmacologic management of cardiogenic shock, according to ACLS guidelines

NOTE: Segue to next slide by introducing Case Study 1.

Slide 4-21 **Case Study 1: Scene Size-up**
▶ Have participants read the case study to themselves. Then provide a synopsis as the slide appears.

Ask: *What is the scene telling you?*
— The problem is probably medical.
— There is one patient.
— This appears to be a safe medical scene so far.
— No need for additional resources at this time.

Ask: *What is the patient telling you?*
— He is in respiratory distress and is potentially unstable.
— He had recent surgery or injury to his foot.
— He is older and possibly may have complicating medical conditions.

Slide 4-22 **Case Study 1: Initial Assessment**
▶ Have participants read the case study to themselves. Then provide a synopsis as the slide appears.
▶ Initial assessment: Look for life threats and intervene if necessary.
▶ Initial impression:
— He is in distress.
— He is in respiratory distress.
— He is showing signs and symptoms of hypoperfusion.
— He is unstable.
▶ Point out that when looking for an initial impression you can also ask:
— What may be wrong with this patient?
— What else could be wrong?
— What should be done next?
▶ This could be a GI bleed; ruptured bowel, appendix, or other structure; sepsis; sickle cell crisis; food poisoning; etc.
▶ Oxygen, IVs, and considering early transport may also be presented.

Slide 4-23   **Case Study 1: OPQRST History**
▶ Point out several items in this history. The healthcare
provider used the classic 1–10 (or 0–10) scale in the
description of severity of dyspnea.
O   Fairly rapid onset
P   Sitting up relieves respiratory distress.
Q   Vague discomfort: "jumping out of my skin"—suggests
skin involvement
R   Does not apply.
S   Dyspnea is severe.
T   Condition is worsening. Syncope suggests hypoperfusion.
▶ Initial impression: shock, possible AMI with failure, sepsis,
anaphylaxis

Slide 4-24   **Case Study 1: SAMPLE History**
▶ Ask for the participants' field impressions. Then tie into the
participants' list of what may be wrong with the patient a
list of differential diagnoses that need to be ruled in/out.
▶ Review the following:
S   Suggests a respiratory problem such as sepsis and
anaphylaxis.
A   None—tends to rule out anaphylaxis—unless this is the
first time for this allergic reaction.
M   Vasotec and Motrin: The Vasotec is an ACE inhibitor
and could inhibit the patient's BP response, or cause
hypotension if taken with alcohol. It may also cause
angioedema of the upper airway. Motrin is associated
with GI bleeds and allergic reactions.
P   Hypertension: Check the patient's normal blood pressure
140/90 on medication. His foot bunionectomy 2 days
ago suggests the patient has been immobile; therefore,
a pulmonary emboli should also be suspected.
L   The patient has eaten, but a blood sugar check may still
be indicated.
E   Since he is older, you should evaluate for an AMI. His
food intake should be evaluated for possible allergic
response.

Slide 4-25   **Case Study 1: Focused Assessment**
▶ Relate this additional information to the participants to
reinforce their field impression.
▶ In order to better understand, compare the signs and
symptoms of anaphylactic shock to the other types of shock
(or classic signs/symptoms).
— This patient is probably suffering from anaphylactic
shock due to the hives and bilateral wheezing.
— Hemorrhagic shock tends to present with cool, pale,
diaphoretic skin and clear lungs.
— Septic shock may involve the lungs, but skin is not
blotchy with hives, so sepsis is probably ruled out.
— Pulmonary emboli may cause shock, but once again
does not usually present with blotchy skin and hives or
wheezes.

SLIDE NO.	SLIDE TITLE/NOTES

Slide 4-26   **General Management of Shock**
▶ Discuss the general principles of shock management.

NOTE: This slide reinforces why it is important for the provider to determine the target organ—differential for the type of shock in the assessment as management is centered around the mechanism.
▶ Giving large amounts of crystalloids is not helpful in anaphylaxis.
▶ Treatment needs to be focused on limiting the allergic/immune response with pharmacologic agents.

Slide 4-27   **Case Study 1: Differential Diagnosis**
▶ Point out that determining the cause of the shock is integral in providing the correct management. Initial impression with differential diagnosis begins with a thorough history and physical exam.
▶ Types of shock are known either by the primary *organ* of dysfunction or by the primary *cause* of dysfunction. History will determine which symptoms began to appear first, possibly indicating which organ is primary.

Slide 4-28   **Specific Management of Anaphylactic Shock**
▶ Controlled fluid administration to challenge preload of the heart and begin to replace fluids lost due to third spacing.
▶ If wheezing with hypotension, a bronchodilator is indicated but with caution in those patients with severe cardiovascular effects.
▶ Epinephrine is indicated in allergic reaction due to its alpha and beta stimulation, along with its ability to limit histamine release from the mast cell.
▶ This drug can be given SC or IV, but IV dose is usually reserved for severe cardiovascular collapse.

NOTE: Epinephrine should be used with caution in those patients > 40 years of age with cardiac history as it increases myocardial oxygen demands.

Slide 4-29   **Case Study 1: Follow-Up**
▶ Some controlled fluid boluses may be administered to replace that lost due to third spacing.
▶ If a patient presents with a mild case of allergic reaction, epinephrine is contraindicated, or if epinephrine does not immediately reverse the reaction, diphenhydramine (Benadryl), a potent antihistamine, can be administered either IV or IM. The onset of action is slower but the duration of action is longer than epinephrine.

Slide 4-30   **Case Study 1: Follow-Up**
Follow-up for Case Study 1

Slide 4-31   **Case Study 2**
▶ You may provide a synopsis of this information after the participants read it to themselves.

Ask: *What is the scene telling you?*
— The problem is probably medical, but trauma cannot be ruled out.
— There is one patient.
— This appears to be a safe scene so far.
— No need for additional resources at this time.

Ask: *What is the patient telling you?*
— He is in respiratory distress and is potentially unstable.
— He is older and possibly may have complicating medical conditions.
— This condition is worse than his normal condition.

Slide 4-32   **Case Study 2: Initial Assessment**
▶ Provide a synopsis and then . . .

Ask: *What treatment needs to be instituted before we move on?*
— Initial assessment: Look for life threats and intervene if necessary.
— Initial impression:
  ▪ He is in distress.
  ▪ He is in respiratory distress.
  ▪ He is showing signs and symptoms of hypoperfusion.
  ▪ He is not mentating well.
  ▪ He is unstable.
▶ Point out that when looking for an initial impression you can also ask:
— What may be wrong with this patient?
— What else could be wrong?
— What should be done next?
▶ This could be an AMI, CHF, COPD, pulmonary emboli, sepsis pneumonia.
▶ Oxygen, monitor, IVs, and considering early transport may also be presented.

Slide 4-33   **Case Study 2: Initial Treatment**
▶ Review information then ask and discuss the following one at a time:
— *What assessment(s) need to be done next?*
— *What history needs to be acquired?*

Slide 4-34   **Case Study 2: OPQRST History**
▶ Give an overview of the information.

Ask: *What is your field impression?*
— This could be an AMI, CHF, COPD, pulmonary emboli, sepsis, pneumonia, GI bleed
▶ Provide positive reinforcement and compile the list of possibilities as differential diagnoses that need to be ruled in/out.
O   Gradual onset.
P   Suggests hypovolemic cause to the hypoperfusion.
Q   Suggest a possible respiratory, cardiac, or GI problem.

    R Does not rule out any possibilities.

    S The pain is not severe, but the elderly may not have good pain perception.

    T Suggests a chronic condition causing his pain.

Slide 4-35   **Case Study 2: SAMPLE History**

▶ Review this information and revisit the list of differential diagnoses.

Ask: *Have any impressions from the previous list been ruled out/in with this information?*

    S Suggests an infectious process.

    A Decreases any suspicion of anaphylaxis.

    M Metformin (glucaphage) is an oral anti-hyperglycemic agent that may cause lactic acidosis. Hypotension and nausea and vomiting may occur if ingested with alcohol. Captopril (Capoten), an ACE inhibitor, may cause hypotension if ingested with alcohol, and is associated with angioedema. Atenolol (Tenormin) is a beta blocker and may not allow normal increases in heart rate and BP to compensate for shock. ASA (aspirin) may be associated with a GI bleed.

    P Diabetes indicates a need to evaluate the blood sugar and possible decreased pain perception; he has a positive cardiac history and should be evaluated for an AMI or CHF. He may have more adhesions and a possible bowel obstruction or his cancer has returned.

    L Suggests GI, concern for blood sugar.

    E Hypovolemia.

Slide 4-36   **Case Study 2: Focused Assessment**

▶ Review this information.

Ask: *What type of shock might this be?*

    — Vital signs suggest septic shock. Drains increase the potential for infection and sepsis along with history of two days illness and fever.

▶ Review the major signs and symptoms with history and findings on physical exam.

▶ Review the prehospital treatment needed for urosepsis and shock.

Slide 4-37   **Case Study 2: Response After Initial Treatment**

▶ Review this information and then ask participants what treatment they recommend.

Slide 4-38   **Case Study 2: Treatment**

▶ The participants have been ordered to provide a dopamine infusion to this septic shock patient after fluid bolus, oxygen, and monitors.

▶ Have participants discuss how to calculate this infusion with the parameters given on the slide. (Slide 4-39 provides the answer.)

▶ OPTION: Have a volunteer go to a board and provide the math for this.

Slide 4-39 **Case Study 2: Dopamine Infusion Calculation**
▶ Brief overview of calculation
— Calculate the dose desired by multiplying patient's weight in kilograms by the amount of micrograms per minute ordered ($80 \times 10 = 800$)
— Calculate the dose available by converting the drug supplied (400 mg) into micrograms (400,000) and instilling it into the solution of 500 ml.
— Calculate how many micrograms in each ml.

$$\frac{\text{Dose Desired}}{\text{Dose Available}} \times \text{Drip Set} = \text{Drops Per Minute}$$

Slide 4-40 **Case Study 2: Follow-Up**
Presents follow-up of Case Study 2.

Slide 4-41 **Summary/Overview—Treatment in Shock**
Emphasize individual treatments for each type of shock.

Slide 4-42 **Summary/Overview—Treatment in Shock (continued)**
Emphasize individual treatments for each type of shock.

Slide 4-43 **Summary Slide for Hypoperfusion Presentation in AMLS**
The healthcare provider must learn to suspect shock, conduct a thorough assessment, recognize the target organ affected and then the type of shock, and provide the specific management needed.

⊞ CHAPTER 5: DYSPNEA, RESPIRATORY DISTRESS, OR RESPIRATORY FAILURE

This interactive lecture includes two case studies. The first case study guides participants through a lower airway emergency and the accompanying pathologies. The second case study is directed at an upper airway problem and the accompanying pathologies. To increase interaction, ask the questions in the notes and allow the participants to answer. Reinforce correct answers. Use the slides to support the answers, but avoid reading the slides to the participants.

SLIDE NO.   **SLIDE TITLE/NOTES**

Slide 5-1   **Dyspnea, Respiratory Distress, or Respiratory Failure**

▶ Difficulty breathing, trouble breathing, respiratory distress are frequent patient complaints.

Ask: *What types of patients do you expect to find. What will they look like?*

Slide 5-2   **Introduction**

▶ Ask participants to give their definition of dyspnea.

▶ Dyspnea is one of the more complex differentials to make, since so many etiologies can have shortness of breath as a sign or symptom.

Slide 5-3   **Anatomy and Physiology**

▶ Review how the structures work together to deliver oxygen to the alveoli and to remove carbon dioxide.

▶ Differentiate between the upper and lower airways.

▶ The larynx is usually the dividing point between the upper and lower airways. Remind participants that it is useful to determine if a problem is in the upper or the lower airway.

Slide 5-4   **Anatomy and Physiology (continued)**

Ask: *Where do you assess for breath sounds?*

— Breath sounds should be assessed bilaterally, contrasted from side to side, at the axilla and at the back.

Slide 5-5   **Minute Volume**

▶ Minute volume is the volume of air exchanged in the lungs in one minute. It is key to evaluate the rate and depth of ventilations. Even though you may not have an exact measurement, the principle of minute volume still applies.

▶ Examples of minute volume:
Ventilatory Rate × Tidal Volume = Minute Volume
12 × 500 cc = 6000 cc
12 × 200 cc = 2400 cc
— The patient is breathing, but the minute volume is inadequate because he is breathing too shallow.
30 × 200 cc = 6000 cc
— The patient is breathing, the minute volume is adequate, but the rate is fast. The work of breathing to maintain an adequate tidal volume has increased.

Ask: *How can you identify increased work of breathing?*

Slide 5-6 **Muscles of Respiration**
▶ Review with participants that accessory muscle use is an indicator of increased work of breathing.
▶ There are both external and internal intercostal muscles that can be utilized to increase ventilatory flow when the patient is in distress.

Slide 5-7 **Important to Note . . .**
▶ Emphasize not using PaO_2 or O_2 saturations as the determining factor. Look at the patient's work of breathing and accessory muscle use. A patient who is laboring to breathe needs intervention regardless of PaO_2 levels.
▶ Transition to the next slide with the following question.

Ask: *Besides use of accessory muscles, what other indicators may be present at the scene to suggest a respiratory problem?*
— Home oxygen devices, medication, piles or bags of tissues, etc.

Slide 5-8 **Scene Size-up**
▶ Follow up answer to previous question. Summarize responses and add any of these the participants did not verbalize.

Slide 5-9 **Assessing Respiratory Compromise**
▶ Review and caution participants about bradypnea and impending respiratory arrest.

Slide 5-10 **Important to Note . . .**
▶ Emphasize aggressive airway management and ventilation in the presence of respiratory failure.

Slide 5-11 **Case Study 1: Scene Size-up**
▶ Allow participants to call out their responses.
▶ Reinforce: The scene is safe, medical in origin, no need for additional resources. She has a history of respiratory problems and is in respiratory distress.
▶ Summarize by reporting that the *initial assessment* indicates a critical patient.

Slide 5-12 **Scene Size-up**
▶ Discuss any factors not brought out in the previous slide. Reinforce chronic vs. acute, multiple problems, and the need for additional assessment, which transitions to the next slide.

Slide 5-13 **Assessment**
▶ Paraphrase the slide.
▶ The signs reinforce the general impression.

Slide 5-14 **Initial Treatment**
▶ Most participants should indicate high-flow O_2 and patient positioning as the first level of treatment.
▶ If no one asks, suggest, "why not a BVM?" Have participants provide a response.

▶ Also ask about the use of a nasal cannula.

▶ After discussion of treatment, ask what the next step should be. This will lead to an OPQRST history.

Slide 5-15 | **Focused History**

▶ Summarize findings.

▶ The question suggests a SAMPLE history be taken.

Slide 5-16 | **Assessment History**

▶ Affirm that the history should include SAMPLE, associated symptoms, and pertinent negatives.

Slide 5-17 | **Focused History—SAMPLE**

▶ Participants should be calling out a variety of diagnoses.

▶ Do not provide the answer yet. Have participants state, based upon their initial suspicions, on which areas of the body they should focus their physical assessment.

▶ The next slide provides answers to the questions.

Slide 5-18 | **Assessment—History**

▶ Review the list. Include any answers not addressed.

Slide 5-19 | **Focused Physical Exam**

▶ Suspicions should be leading toward asthma, COPD, or CHF.

▶ Have participants defend their diagnoses.

▶ If there is a consensus answer, suggest other diagnoses. Have participants critique/consider these potentials.

Slide 5-20 | **Causes of Dyspnea**

▶ As you progress through the causes of dyspnea relate them to the case study.

▶ Allow participants to read the slide. Reinforce any points listed below.

— Asthma

— She has a known history.

— She is on asthma medications.

— She uses an inhaler and oral steroids.

— She is wheezing.

▶ As a differential in the patient with dyspnea, the respiratory system itself could be the culprit.

Slide 5-21 | **Causes of Dyspnea**

▶ Relate the causes of dyspnea to Case Study 1.

— CHF: She has wheezing, JVD, and a nocturnal onset, so CHF should be considered. However, she does not take any of the medications associated with CHF or have pedal edema, which decrease the chance that this is CHF.

— Cardiac tamponade: She has JVD, which can be caused by cardiac tamponade, but she does not have any of the other symptoms, so this diagnosis is not likely.

Ask: *Which diagnosis best fits the patient presentation?*

— Probably cardiac asthma/acute pulmonary edema. But asthma cannot be ruled out.

Ask: *What could be the treatments? How do they compare?*
— Treatment for CHF may include oxygen, Lasix (furosemide), nitroglycerin, morphine sulfate, CPAP, albuterol for bronchospasm (can cause cardiac dysrhythmias).
— Treatment for asthma may include oxygen, beta-adrenergic agents such as albuterol, sub-q epinephrine, terbutaline, steroids or anticholinergic agents (Atrovent), magnesium sulfate.

▶ These treatments must be weighed carefully if she has a primary cardiac problem. The beta adrenergic agents or magnesium sulfate may worsen her cardiac condition.

▶ If her primary condition is asthma, Lasix may worsen the condition by drying the secretions.

▶ The best approach: Begin slowly with the agents that have the least side effects and monitor the patient for response and confirmation of diagnosis.

Slide 5-22   Final Impression

▶ Most likely, the patient is experiencing her first episode of CHF resulting from an MI.

▶ This episode is different from her prior episodes of dyspnea. It is described as being worse, and she has chest tightness not previously experienced. Remember that older female patients often do not feel typical ischemic cardiac chest pain. Other signs and symptoms consistent with CHF include PND, JVD, and poor lung sounds (wheezing and diminished).

▶ CHF patients usually also have a history of hypertension. She may have asthma, but wheezing is also possible with CHF. There was no relief from three self-administered inhaler doses.

▶ JVD in the absence of peripheral edema suggests that the heart failure is not chronic. She may be developing a right-sided heart failure component.

▶ Have participants discuss and justify. They do not all have to agree with each other.

Slide 5-23   Case Study 2: Scene Size-up

▶ Allow participants to call out their responses.

▶ Reinforce: The scene is safe, medical in origin, the patient is critical, additional resources may be needed if initial response was at BLS level.

▶ Summarize by reporting that the *initial assessment* indicates a critical patient.

▶ Again, participants should respond with a few potential diagnoses.

▶ Initial actions include an initial assessment, continue BVM with O_2 if necessary, intubate if possible, establish C-spine precautions, EKG, IV.

Slide 5-24 — Considerations

- Discuss any factors not brought out by the participants.
- Reinforce chronic vs. acute, multiple problems, and the need for immediate intervention.
- Additional assessment may occur as patient is being managed, which transitions to the next slide.
- Question whether C-spine immobilization is indicated. Discuss unknown cause, possible trauma since she is at the beach. No immobilization is also an option if questioning does not reveal trauma.

Slide 5-25 — Initial Assessment

- Reposition the head, have high-flow oxygen and BVM ready for use.
- There may be a response of utilizing the Heimlich maneuver. This would be reasonable, only after a repositioning of the head.

Slide 5-26 — Immediate Actions
Review steps.

Slide 5-27 — Initial Assessment

- Review actions with participants and progress to the following.
- Considerations include:
  - Ventilate the patient with high-flow O_2.
  - Begin assembly of equipment for rapid transport.
  - Place a cervical collar and immobilize patient to backboard.
  - Monitor patient and consider intravenous access.
  - Perform a rapid physical assessment of the unconscious patient.
- A form of surgical airway or needle cricothyrotomy may be suggested, although it should be pointed out that there is some air exchange with a basic airway maneuver.

Slide 5-28 — Additional Steps
Review steps.

Slide 5-29 — Initial Assessment

- Review with participants.
- Impression—probable anaphylaxis. The participants should be asking about lung sounds. If not, prompt them for a response.
- Progress to complete a differential diagnosis. Have participants rationalize their answers.
- Next steps include establishing baseline vital signs (medication therapy may be premature at this point, without having a complete picture of the patient presentation).

Slide 5-30 — Assessment—History
Review.

Slide 5-31 **Focused Exam**
- ▶ The anaphylaxis diagnosis is more justified at this point.
- ▶ Epinephrine is a reasonable response.

Slide 5-32 **Focused History**
- ▶ Reassess for response; suggest second dose of epinephrine if no response to first dose.
- ▶ Diphenhydramine should be considered.

Slide 5-33 **Treatment, Continuing Assessment**
- ▶ Review findings and implications.

Slide 5-34 **Causes of Dyspnea**
- ▶ Foreign body: There was evidence of ingestion; it was a sudden onset.
- ▶ Infection: She has no fever, sudden onset not gradual.
- ▶ Anaphylaxis: Sudden onset, wheezing rash, responds to epinephrine.

Slide 5-35 **Causes of Dyspnea**
- ▶ Angioedema: She has swelling of the hands and airway.
- ▶ No evidence of others, although irritant exposure cannot be ruled out.

Slide 5-36 **Causes of Dyspnea**
- ▶ No evidence of these diseases. She had a sudden onset.

Slide 5-37 **Causes of Dyspnea**
- ▶ No evidence of these factors since it was a sudden onset.

Slide 5-38 **Additional Considerations**
- ▶ Given the information, the patient probably is having an allergic reaction and the anaphylaxis protocol is indicated.

Slide 5-39 **Final Considerations**
- ▶ Discuss the final impression. Address the issue of other causes of the anaphylaxis.
- ▶ Address need for previous exposure prior to anaphylactic response.

Slide 5-40 **Summary**
- ▶ Emphasize the priority of dyspnea.

▦ CHAPTER 6: CHEST PAIN

SLIDE NO.	SLIDE TITLE/NOTES

Slide 6-1 **Chest Pain**
- ▶ Chest pain immediately invokes thoughts of acute coronary syndrome or AMI.
- ▶ However, there are many other things that can cause chest pain.

Slide 6-2 **Introduction**
- ▶ Up to 5% of all patients who turn out to have acute myocardial infarction are initially discharged from the Emergency Department even after EKG, chest radiograph, and lab evaluations.
- ▶ Because of this, every chest pain is initially treated as a serious condition.

Slide 6-3 **Anatomy and Physiology**
- ▶ Emphasize chest pain can originate outside of the chest.

Slide 6-4 **Thoracic Structures**
- ▶ Any disease process that affects structures lying within the thoracic cavity can produce chest pain.

Slide 6-5 **Types of Chest Pain**
- ▶ Somatic: pain that originates from nerve fibers located in the skin or parietal pleura
- ▶ Visceral: pain that originates from pain fibers in organs or the visceral pleura

Slide 6-6 **Assessment Priorities**
- ▶ History and physical exam will be key to identifying the cause of chest pain.

Slide 6-7 **Focused History**
Summarize.

Slide 6-8 **Management Priorities**
Emphasize timely treatment and prompt transport.

Slide 6-9 **General Management Priorities**
Review.

Slide 6-10 **Case Study 1: Scene Size-up**
- ▶ EMS is responding to street corner for a patient complaining of chest pain.
- ▶ Ask the participants to size up the scene.

Ask: *Is the patient stable or unstable?*
— Unstable

Ask: *What stands out in the scenario?*
— Answers should include: scene safety, difficulty breathing, AMI, pale diaphoretic skin.

NOTE: Do not proceed to the next slide until participants interact.

Slide 6-11 **Scene Size-up**
▶ This slide answers previous slide.
▶ Chest pain and dyspnea on exertion are symptoms of possible cardiac or respiratory related conditions.

Slide 6-12 **Initial Assessment**
Ask: *Is this patient stable or unstable?*
— Unstable

Ask: *What stands out in the scenario?*
— Respiratory rate is fast.
— Unable to speak in more than 2–3 word sentences
— Accessory muscle use
— Lung sounds are bilaterally diminished.

Slide 6-13 **Treatment**
▶ Initiate treatment immediately while assessment continues.

Slide 6-14 **Focused History**
▶ Allow participants to read the slide. Ask about Beck's Triad.
▶ Discuss Beck's Triad: Consists of distended neck veins, hypotension, and muffled heart sounds and is associated with cardiac tamponade.
▶ Refresh participants on the patient's symptoms. (This patient had distended neck veins, but his BP was adequate. Heart tones were not presented.)
▶ Therefore, additional history and presentation are key.
▶ History of pericarditis may contribute to the presentation. History of an AMI, diabetes, and COPD are also factors. Patient also describes a squeezing pain and an increased tightness with a deep breath.
▶ Based on these findings, AMI and a developing pneumothorax must be considered.

Slide 6-15 **Focused History**
▶ Have participants discuss their suspicions.

Slide 6-16 **Considerations**
▶ Based on all these factors, this patient must be a candidate for rapid workup and urgent transport.

Slide 6-17 **Causes of Chest Pain**
▶ Discuss this patient's presentation and place him in the potentially life-threatening category.
▶ Describe the different disease process.
▶ Have the class come up with differential diagnosis.
▶ Discussion may include the following.
— AMI—Previous history, may not present with typical signs and symptoms due to diabetes; pain is not usual AMI pain.
— Unstable angina—Possible, pain is not consistent with usual presentation, not likely.
— Aortic dissection—Pain is not tearing, so not likely.
— Esophageal rupture—Pain is not sharp and steady. Pain is isolated to heart, so not likely.

— Cardiac tamponade—Pain is consistent as are early signs of shock; possible.

— Tension pneumothorax—Distended neck veins and difficulty breathing present, but equal breath sounds tend to rule this one out.

Slide 6-18   **Detailed Physical Exam**

Ask: *How does the secondary assessment lead you toward supporting your diagnosis?*

— Equal breath sounds continue to rule out tension pneumothorax.

— Muffled heart tones support cardiac tamponade.

— Abdominal causes not likely.

Slide 6-19   **Overview**

Ask: *Has your decision about the diagnosis changed?*

▶ Have participants defend their diagnosis.

Slide 6-20   **Overview**

▶ Discuss how participants may have been mislead by symptoms.

Slide 6-21   **Signs of Cardiac Tamponade**

▶ Discuss Beck's Triad.

Slide 6-22   **Cardiac Tamponade**

▶ Allow participants to read. Point out keys (Beck's Triad).

▶ Keys are in recognizing the signs and symptoms and prompt transport to definitive care for a pericardiocentesis.

Slide 6-23   **Case Study 2: Scene Size-up**

▶ EMS is responding to a residence for a pregnant patient complaining of chest discomfort.

Ask: *Is the scene secure?*
Is the patient stable or unstable?

— Scene is secure.

— Patient is unstable.

Ask: *What stands out in the scenario?*

— Pain with breathing

— Pregnancy

NOTE: Do not proceed to the next slide until participants interact.

Slide 6-24   **Initial Assessment**

Ask: *Why is this patient's condition serious?*

— The patient is disoriented.

— Abnormal breath sounds

— Increased heart rate

— Skin is cool and diaphoretic.

— Slow respiratory rate

Ask: *What is going on at this point?*

— Asthma, pulmonary emboli, shock, foreign body, etc.

Ask: *Is it too early to make a diagnosis?*

Ask: *What is your initial treatment?*
— Oxygen, turn her on her left side, monitor, transport, IV, ongoing assessment

Slide 6-25   **Focused History**
Ask: *What has changed your impression?*
— Patient felt faint and fell, longer 2-hour onset, dull pain in her chest, pain radiates to her lower back.

Ask: *What differentials have you added?*
— Chest and abdominal trauma list, head trauma

Slide 6-26   **Focused History**
Ask: *What has changed your impression?*
— She was asymptomatic prior to falling.

Ask: *What diagnosis have you added or changed?*
— Eliminate asthma, others?

Slide 6-27   **Causes of Chest Pain**
Ask: *Does the patient have a potentially life-threatening condition or a non-life-threatening condition?*
▶ Participants must defend their answers.
▶ Review the list and have participants discuss which they think she might have.

Slide 6-28   **Detailed Physical Exam**
Ask: *Has your decision about the diagnosis changed?*
▶ Have participants defend their diagnoses.
— A pneumothorax should be on the list due to diminished breath sounds on the left.
— A murmur and S3 may indicate cardiac involvement.

Slide 6-29   **Second Set of Vitals**
▶ The increased respiratory rate may be due to the decreased breath sounds, or hypoxia.

Slide 6-30   **Possible Causes of Tachycardia**
▶ Discuss which of these is likely for this patient and why.
— Pulmonary embolism—Yes, pregnant females are more likely to have PE due to the hypercoagulation state they are in and due to venous pooling in the lower legs.
— Pneumonia—Not likely due to onset. The problem started after a fall, with no evidence of illness prior to that point.
— Tension pneumothorax—Not likely due to breath sounds and adequate BP. Monitor for tension pneumothorax because pneumothorax is possible.
— Anxiety—Yes, a diagnosis of exclusion.
— Pain—Yes, she has chest discomfort.
— Hypoxia—Yes, she has altered breath sounds which may contribute to hypoxia.
— Supine hypotensive syndrome—Yes, keep her positioned off her back.

	SLIDE NO.	SLIDE TITLE/NOTES

Slide 6-31   **Overview**
Ask: *Has your decision about the diagnosis changed?*
▸ Have participants defend their diagnoses.

Slide 6-32   **Considerations**
▸ Review.

Slide 6-33   **Overview**
▸ Dyspnea occurs in 85% of the cases.
▸ Tachypnea occurs in 90% of the cases.
▸ Syncope occurs in 10% of the cases. Even though it is rare, it is a significant finding.
▸ Diaphoresis may occur and worsen with signs of shock.
▸ S2 murmur and right-sided S3 occurs due to the increased pulmonic valve closure in 50% of the cases.
▸ Localized wheezing may be present.
▸ Because she is pregnant, pulmonary emboli should be a consideration.

Slide 6-34   **Pulmonary Embolism**
▸ Discuss the history of risk factors, but emphasize 20% of the patients will have no pre-existing history of risk factors.
▸ Pulmonary embolism may produce chest pain. Patients may complain of sharp, pleuritic chest pain, tachycardia, and tachypnea.
▸ If greater than one half of the pulmonary vasculature is involved, this is a serious, life-threatening condition. The patient will present with shock symptoms, dyspnea, and hypoxia.
▸ The patients may have crackles or a pleural rub.

Slide 6-35   **Acute Myocardial Infarction**
▸ History—An AMI should be suspected in those males greater than 30 years old, and in females greater than 40 years old, especially with positive risk factors for this disease.
▸ Types of pain—Review classic signs and symptoms and then highlight that older patient, diabetics, and females sometimes present without chest pain.
▸ Highlight the associated symptoms. Physical findings are usually not helpful in the diagnosis.
▸ Treatment includes: oxygen, IV, and monitor(s); early administration of aspirin; vasoactive pain management with nitrates and morphine. An early 12-lead ECG needs to be done. A normal ECG can be seen in many ischemic cascades.

Slide 6-36   **Signs and Symptoms of an AMI**
Review.

Slide 6-37   **12-lead Interpretation**
▸ Allow participants to review and summarize.

Slide 6-38   **Unstable Angina**
- ▶ Emphasize like an AMI but occur more often with exertion and are relieved promptly by rest or nitroglycerin. Pain is usually short, 5–15 minutes. Treat as a possible AMI.

Slide 6-39   **Aortic Dissection**
- ▶ The classic patient is a hypertensive male of 40–70 years of age.
- ▶ Ehlers-Danlos syndrome is an inherited disorder of connective tissue that makes the vessels fragile. Aortic dissection may occur in younger patients with this disorder.
- ▶ Marfan's syndrome is a hereditary disorder of connective tissue that creates a tall, lean body with long extremities (fingers and toes). The aorta is dilated and susceptible to dissection.
- ▶ Pain is usually a tearing pain that is severe at first, then becomes intermittent. The symptoms will vary depending on location of the dissection:
  - — Aortic arch: Carotid and subclavian area produce a stroke-like presentation or a pulseless arm. In extreme cases cardiac tamponade may occur.
  - — Descending thoracic/abdominal/iliac aorta areas may dissect into the arteries that perfuse individual organs.
- ▶ Treatment depends on location and symptoms and may be either medical or surgical.

Slide 6-40   **Perforation of the Esophagus**
- ▶ Is usually associated with sudden forceful vomiting, coughing, or with procedures such as NG tube placement.
- ▶ The pain is sharp, steady in the anterior, posterior, and epigastric regions and may radiate to the neck.
- ▶ Symptoms include dysphagia and hemoptysis with pleural friction rub, fever, tachycardia, tachypnea, hypotension.
- ▶ Treatment is geared to supporting the patient with aggressive fluid resuscitation and management for sepsis.
- ▶ High mortality rate

Slide 6-41   **Pericarditis**
- ▶ Pericarditis is an inflammation of the pericardial sac that surrounds the heart.
- ▶ The chest pain is steady, burning, and retrosternal and may radiate into the back, neck, scapula, or jaw.
- ▶ It may worsen with deep breathing and pulsate with each beat of the heart. It is worse upon lying down—improves with sitting up or leaning forward.
- ▶ A pericardial rub may be heard, often heard best when the patient leans forward.
- ▶ There may be ST-segment elevation or depression throughout leads, without localization.

Slide 6-42   **ECG Findings with Pericarditis**
Review.

	SLIDE NO.	SLIDE TITLE/NOTES

Slide 6-43 **Gastrointestinal Disorders**

▶ GI disorders can cause chest pain. This is because the sensory nerve fibers are shared between many abdominal structures and the thorax.

▶ They usually present with retrosternal burning, similar to AMI. Pain may radiate to the throat, and patients may have heartburn or indigestion.

▶ It is usually worse at night when they lie down or lean forward.

▶ They may have pain on palpation while an AMI patient usually will not.

Slide 6-44 **Mitral Valve Prolapse**

▶ Elastic mitral valve expands into the left atrium during systole. This causes episodes of chest pain due to stretching of the chordae tendonae and papillary muscles.

▶ Patient symptoms include vertigo, dyspnea, palpitations, and syncope. Systolic murmur (click) and cardiac dysrhythmias may be found.

▶ Most patients are asymptomatic.

Slide 6-45 **Summary**

▶ Ask for questions and summarize.

SLIDE NO. | **SLIDE TITLE/NOTES**

Slide 7-1 | **Altered Mental Status**
▶ AMS is a sign of physiological instability.
▶ It is not a disease, but can be an ominous sign of an underlying life threat. The assessment and management focus is to develop an initial impression and move to "rule in/rule out" possibilities. While gathering historical information, narrow the focus to probabilities to determine a differential field diagnosis.
▶ Focus on the difference between the life threats and non-life threats.

Slide 7-2 | **Pathophysiology**
▶ The majority of AMS and comatose states are explained with reference to dysfunction of the RAS and/or the cerebrum.
▶ Cerebrum maintains a state of awareness; the RAS maintains states of arousal/awareness; that is, the lights are on but no one is home.
▶ The cerebrum is the awakeness—the lights are on; the RAS is the awareness—no one is home.
▶ A person with an intact RAS and two cerebral hemispheres has full orientation.
▶ Dysfunction of both cerebral hemispheres means serious alteration in mentation.
▶ If one hemisphere is dysfunctional, the patient is conscious/aware but has behavioral changes and/or loss of neurological ability.
— Example: CVA where damage in one hemisphere exhibits confusion and impaired motor/sensory on the opposite side of infarct.

Slide 7-3 | **Pathophysiology**
▶ The RAS obtains sensory input from environment on a constant basis.
▶ It filters the necessary input for a response from hemispheres. (e.g., If you take off your watch every night at bedtime, generally you don't pay attention to the action. However, if the watch breaks and falls to floor, RAS.)
▶ It sends message to thalamus that an action is needed. Thalamus sends message to various parts of the cerebral cortex for action. Motor area may allow for picking up pieces. Association areas may allow for emotional response. We can have good awareness with functioning RAS and one cerebral hemisphere.
▶ Since RAS receives and relays information, any breakdown in RAS blocks transmission of stimuli. If information doesn't reach cortex, decreased awareness can result, even if cerebrum intact.

SLIDE NO.	SLIDE TITLE/NOTES

Slide 7-4   **Pathophysiology**

▶ The cerebrum has unmylenated fibers, therefore slower impulse movement to accommodate time for thalamus to interpret RAS impulses. The association areas are the most fascinating.

▶ They interpret sensory input from the RAS for response/action. Higher levels of thinking—ability to analyze, reason, judgment, mood, conscience—separate us from other animals.

▶ Children under 3, who have decreased stimulus to the RAS and related association areas may have poor social development, decreased critical thinking, and potential academic difficulty.

▶ Right and left hemisphere damage will show different signs and symptoms in patients.

Slide 7-5   **The Cerebrum**

▶ Knowing CNS anatomy and physiology and their relationship to signs and symptoms guides us to more rapid identification of underlying etiology and management. Motor speech area has Wernicke area. This area is responsible for comprehension and understanding of spoken and written word.

▶ The Brocca area is responsible for physical speech and forming words. If damaged, there is a communication problem and difficulty eliciting history.

— For example, in patients with stroke, if Brocca area is damaged they can understand your commands/questions, but are unable to answer you, resulting in frustration, unintentional anger. If the Wernicke area is damaged they will not be able to understand your commands and may babble words that appear not to make sense.

▶ Frontal lobe is responsible for cognition and intellect, higher learning, thinking outside the box. During 1930–50s, area of brain where lobotomy performed to sever neuronal pathway in patients exhibiting bizarre behavior. The motor area controls skeletal muscle.

▶ Damaged respiratory muscles can be life-threatening. Premotor area stores motor skills of repetition (e.g., typing, playing the piano). If damaged, this is one area that can be reprogrammed and skills relearned through occupational therapy.

▶ Sensory association area interprets somatic input—temperature, pressure, texture, size. For example, it helps interpret the difference between a coin and a key as you reach into your pocket.

▶ Visual association area interprets and stores information from past visual experience. It helps differentiate between a face and a flower. If damaged, a patient may be unable to recognize or comprehend the difference between pill bottles, which leads to toxicity.

Slide 7-6   **Structural and Metabolic Alterations**

▶ Understanding relationship between structural and metabolic damages and AMS allows for rapid identification of underlying cause of AMS and treatment. Structural and metabolic alterations generally affect the cerebral hemispheres and awakeness.

▶ Some structural or traumatic injuries may involve RAS and decrease awareness. Structural emergencies are more sudden in onset; patients have unequal pupils and increased ICP.

▶ May affect the RAS.

▶ Metabolic alterations affect the brain indirectly. Imbalance in sodium, calcium, thiamine. Damage by either causes AMS.

Slide 7-7   **AMS Assessment**

▶ Application of knowledge of anatomy and physiology and systematic assessment processes are imperative for management of patients with chief complaints of AMS.

Slide 7-8   **Focused History**

▶ Assessment of OPQRST and SAMPLE allow for progression from possibilities to probabilities and differential field diagnosis.

Slide 7-9   **Differential Field Diagnosis—AMS Environmental Factors—Heat/Cold**

▶ Heat exhaustion is most often the result of exertion in hot environment with high humidity. This results in loss of fluids and electrolytes causing dehydration.

▶ Signs and symptoms are tachycardia; tachypnea; cool, clammy, diaphoretic skin; abdominal cramping; normal BP; ataxia; confusion; and agitation.

▶ Core temperature generally 98°F (37°C). Hypothermia core temperatures of 84–94°F (30–34°C).

▶ Hypothalamus unable to warm body. Patient exhibits hypoxia, coma, bradycardia with J (Osborn) wave that follows the QRS.

▶ Heat stroke exhibits core temperatures of greater than 105°F (40°C). Hypothalamus unable to cool resulting cerebral edema; confusion to coma; hot, dry skin; tachypnea is early sign, bradypnea late sign; decreased BP.

▶ AMS is significant and is a life-threatening emergency.

▶ Management is oxygen, ventilation, oral fluids if conscious, core rectal temperature, handle gently. Remove from environment and cool/warm to normal body temperature.

▶ Hypothermia and heat stroke may require peritoneal lavage.

Slide 7-10 **AMS Environmental Factors—Sanitation/Nutrition**

▶ Chronic alcoholism precipitates hypoglycemia, GI bleeds, esophageal varices, subdural hematomas, diabetic emergencies, electrolyte imbalances, and thiamine deficiency.

Slide 7-11   **Differential Field Diagnosis—Thiamine Deficiency**
- Thiamine deficiency is vitamin B[1] deficiency from improper diet. Thiamine metabolizes carbohydrates to create ATP energy for cell activity.
- Decreased levels cause brain edema and decreased cerebral perfusion. Wernicke—appears hypoglycemic or intoxicated, discongugate gaze, ataxia, confusion, lethargy, nystagmus (ocular paralysis).
- Korsakoff's syndrome exhibits amnesia, hallucinations.
- Assessment includes poor living conditions, alcohol intoxication, diminished cognition. Abdomen evaluation for wasting, distention, ascites.

Slide 7-12   **Management of Thiamine Deficiency**
- Routine medical care. If able to obtain IV access, can give 50 mg thiamine IVP for rapid infusion effects and 50 mg IM for slower effects.

Slide 7-13   **Differential Diagnosis—Thyroid Disorders—Lethargy**
- The thyroid gland regulates the metabolic rate through the release of hormones in the blood.
- Hypothyroidism results from decreased release of thyroid hormone as a result of pituitary gland dysfunction. It exhibits signs ans symptoms of decreased cognition, decreased memory, ataxia, weakness, weight gain, intolerance to cold, edema of hands and feet, moon face, bradycardia, and CHF related to decreased CO. Meds taken: Synthroid, levothryoxine.
- Hyperthyroidism exhibits agitation, psychosis, hyperactivity, weight loss, infection, emotional stress.
- Often taking Propacil, Tapazole, iodine, and weight loss medications.
- Management includes routine medical care, emotional support.
- For hyperthyroidism check blood glucose level for hypoglycemia and dehydration. Fluids 20 cc/kg and D_{50} may be appropriate due to energy and fluid consumption related to hyperactivity.
- Maintain body temperature. Beta blockers may be given for hyperthyroidism.
- Hepatic encephalopathy—liver cleanses blood and converts ammonia into urea. If liver not functioning, blood bypasses it and ammonia levels increase to toxic levels in brain causing seizure and ICP.
- Assess for history of alcohol, cirrhosis, hepatitis, spider angiomas, ascites secondary to portal hypertension, yellow sclera, and fector hepaticus (musty breath odor).

7-14   **Differential Field Diagnosis—Measurable Abnormal Findings**
- Hypoglycemia presents with low blood glucose level of < 60 mg/dl with signs and symptoms or < 50 mg/dl without signs and symptoms. Patients have taken insulin, not eaten,

or have been ill with flu, infection, or overexertion. Patient presentation is lethargic; cool, clammy, diaphoretic skin; acute onset; full, rapid pulses; normal blood pressure; abdominal pain with electrolyte imbalance; history of obesity.

▶ Hyperglycemia reveals blood glucose levels > 300 mg/dl. Insulin not transporting glucose causing accumulation in cells. Increased blood glucose level increases osmotic pressure and draws water from interstitial and intracellular area causing cellular dehydration. They have eaten, not enough insulin present. Anaerobic metabolism occurs in an effort to return pH to normal by excreting CO_2. Ketones are byproduct and result in fruity breath odor. Sunken orbits related to dehydration, confusion, hunger, thirst, Kussmaul's respirations. Weak, rapid pulses, poor skin turgor, pallor.

▶ Delayed capillary refill related to dehydration, slow healing wounds, distal neuropathy, poor peripheral perfusion, scarring of fingers, lower extremity amputations/prosthesis, abdominal cramping due to fluid shifts, later stages low blood pressure. Increased urination at approximately > 180 mg/dl as kidney cannot reabsorb excess glucose and it spills into urine, exacerbating dehydration. Exhibits signs and symptoms of dehydration, tachycardia, low BP, dry mucous membranes, etc.

▶ Different ethnic groups may compensate differently. For example, Native Americans can exhibit 300–500 mg/dl and be asymptomatic. Signs and symptoms of hypoglycemia may be present, but may display 300–500 mg/dl.

Slide 7-15   Differential Field Diagnosis—Miscellaneous Findings
▶ Related to diabetes and/or renal disease
▶ Assess for dialysis shunts, last visit to dialysis, scarred fingers from blood letting to check blood glucose level, and polyuria, polydispia, polyphagia.

Slide 7-16   Management of Diabetic Complications
▶ Hyperglycemic hyperosmolar nonketonic coma—produces insulin, but not enough to meet cellular demands.
▶ Fluid shifts from extravascular to intravascular spaces causing cellular dehydration in brain, electrolyte loss, and behavior changes.
▶ Patient will be dehydrated, but have enough insulin to transport
▶ Glucose. No acidosis, Kussmaul or ketone odors. No anaerobic metabolism.
▶ Patients with this condition are resistant to insulin.

Slide 7-17   Management of Diabetic Complications—Hypoglycemia
▶ Assessment that leads to management includes:
— Scene size-up looking for syringes, insulin containers, glucometer, prosthesis, or assistive devices

    — Physical exam includes thorough neurological exam as symptoms mimic stroke and seizure. Determine if onset was gradual or sudden

    — Associated disease processes include renal and cardiac anomalies.

Slide 7-18   **Diabetic Management—Hypoglycemia**

▶ Regardless of the type of diabetic complication, maintenance of the patient's ABCs are a must. Prevent aspiration of gastric contents while the patient has an altered mental status; provide good minute volume and oxygenation if necessary. For the patient who is maintaining his or her own airway patency and is not vomiting, delay endotracheal intubation until the underlying condition is reversed.

▶ Give 18-gauge IV of isotonic crystalloid and use of 50% dextrose if the blood sugar is < 40 mg/dl with altered mental status.

▶ For those with confusion without decreased mental status, oral ingestion of food, drink, or instant glucose is recommended.

▶ If a peripheral IV cannot be established, 1 mg of glucagon may be given IM. This frees the stored glycogen from the liver and increases the overall blood glucose level. This may be ineffective if stored glycogen has been depleted. Peak effect should be in 10-20 minutes.

▶ The malnourished hypoglycemic patient should have simultaneous administration of thiamine (Vitamin B[1]) as it assists in glucose conversion.

▶ If a hypoglycemic patient does not rapidly improve with 50% dextrose, re-evaluate for the need for thiamine. The dose is 100 mg and can be given IV or IM.

Slide 7-19   **Diabetic Management—DKA/HHNC**

▶ For those hyperglycemic patients (whether DKA or HHNC), dehydration is very common and 20 ml/kg bolus (according to protocol) may be given judiciously.

▶ BUT REMEMBER—most diabetics present with many medical co-existing problems.

    — Most commonly—cardiac and renal

    — Fluid boluses should be given with frequent re-evaluation.

Slide 7-20   **Common Causes of Acid-Base Disturbance**

▶ Assessment of these disturbances include:

    — Scene size-up evaluation for history of use of cigarettes, multiple medications, drug paraphernalia, evidence of diabetes or renal failure, poor living conditions, malnutrition.

    — Facial affect in acidosis will be lethargy, alkalosis, hyperactivity.

    — Assessment of ABCs includes evaluation of respiratory patterns and administration of oxygen and/or ventilation.

    — Chief complaint of lethargy, weakness, confusion, kidney dialysis, COPD, chest pain in acidosis

— Chief complaints of muscular spasticity, ataxia, numbness and tingling in extremities, dizziness, diarrhea or vomiting prior to illness, and inappropriate behavior in alkalosis

— SAMPLE history includes usage of other medications, last oral intake, and history of vomiting. Assess for gradual or sudden onset to determine severity.

— Physical exam includes evaluation of mucosa for hydration, carpal pedal spasm (alkalosis), and delay in capillary refill (alkalosis). Vital signs may vary.

  ▪ In acidosis pulses remain normal or slightly elevated and as symptoms worsen become weaker and slower.

  ▪ Alkalosis typically presents with elevated pulses.

▶ Definitive treatment may not be accomplished in the field and may be directed at management of life threats only.

— For respiratory acidosis and alkalosis oxygen and ventilation are appropriate.

— Respiratory acidosis may include bronchodilators for COPD and naloxone for overdose. If fluid accumulates in lungs from pneumonia or infectious disease, the patient can be placed in High Fowlers to allow gravity to help drain fluid and improve gas exchange.

— BVM can be used to assist excretion of CO_2.

— In respiratory alkalosis, coach the patient to decrease respirations to help decrease pH by closing mouth and breathing through nose.

— Treat cardiac dysrhythmias per AHA recommendations. In metabolic acidosis administration of bicarbonate IVP 1 mEq/kg may be appropriate.

— IV therapy should remain TKO in an effort not to dilute electrolyte concentrations. Arterial blood gases (ABGs) should be obtained for more definitive diagnosis and management.

Slide 7-21   Assessment of Acid-Base Disturbances

▶ Two of the major contributors to acid-base imbalance are disturbances in sodium and calcium.

▶ Sodium—primary cation in extracellular fluid. Distributes water and also is responsible for protection, waste removal, and thermoregulation.

▶ Normal values are 135-145 mEq/l. Hypernatremia increases intracellular osmolarity causing cellular dehydration.

— The shrinkage of cells affects the size of the brain cells and can actually decrease the size of the brain itself. This condition alters nerve depolarization causing irritability and seizures.

— As brain vessels shrink there is greater risk of rupture.

— Hyponatremia causes extracellular shifts into intracellular spaces causing edema.

— The edema results in increased ICP and decreased cerebral perfusion.

— Typical symptoms include headache, stupor and seizure, pathologic respiratory patterns, facial palsy/droop, tongue deviation, aphasia, vision and pupil changes, and NVD.

— May be taking potassium supplements, diuretics, digitalis, beta blockers, and thiazides.

▶ Calcium—a cation stored in bones and teeth that maintains cell stability. This cation regulates calcium entry in cell, blood clotting mechanisms, nerve and muscle impulses, myocardial contraction.

▶ Normal ranges are 9–10 mg/dl.

▶ Hypercalcemia—increases permeability to sodium and decreases electrical impulse conduction diminishing CNS function.

— Decreased neurotransmission causes seizures, muscle weakness, decrease myocardial automaticity leading to severe heart blocks, decreased cardiac output, and decreased cerebral perfusion.

— Symptoms include hyperactive parathyroid (which regulates calcium), shortened QT and ST segments, shallow respirations, chest pain, syncopal episodes.

— Hypocalcaemia allows sodium to enter cell and increase depolarization.

— Patients exhibit tetany, convulsions, prolonged QT and ST segments, decreased myocardial contractions, pulmonary congestion, poor peripheral perfusion.

▶ Field management focuses on managing life threats and rapid transport for definitive diagnosis and treatment.

Slide 7-22   **Differential Field Diagnosis—Pain**

▶ Pain is also used in differential diagnosis. Chest pain is considered to be cardiac related until proven otherwise.

▶ Chest pain can also be a result of electrolyte imbalance and diabetes.

▶ Syncopal episodes that occur when a patient is sitting or at rest are cardiac in nature until proven otherwise.

▶ History of flu, fever, taking antibiotics, pain, and stiff neck can be related to meningitis. Patients will complain of being light and sound sensitive.

— Signs of meningeal inflammation include flexion of the head that causes neck pain and a reflexive flexion of the hip and knees (Brudzinski's sign) and flexion of the extremities with pain and resistance on subsequent straightening (Kernig's sign).

Slide 7-23   **Differential Field Diagnosis—Cranial Infection**

▶ Similar to stroke with visual disturbances, pupil dysfunction, facial droop, swallowing difficulty, tongue deviation, weakness in extremities, ataxia, incontinence

▶ BP is typically normal to elevated.

▶ Irregular respiratory patterns from ICP, history of headache, fever, sinus infection, hemiplegia, hemiparesis, visual deficit

▸ Tachycardia from hypermetabolic state with hot, dry, flushed skin

Slide 7-24   **Cranial Infections—Meningitis**
▸ Since the cranial vault is closed, inflammation causes increase in ICP. ICP obstructs flow of cerebrospinal fluid decreasing nutrition to brain.

Slide 7-25   **Cranial Infections—Signs and Symptoms of Meningitis**

Slide 7-26   **Cranial Infections—Encephalitis**

Slide 7-27   **Cranial Infections—Signs and Symptoms of Encephalitis**
▸ Infection of the brain itself:
— Occurs elsewhere in the body and finds its way to the brain via the peripheral nerves and blood vessels.
— Can cause coma if involvement includes the RAS.
— Rabies is an underlying cause.
— Difficult to distinguish from meningitis in the field.

Slide 7-28   **Cranial Infections—Signs and Symptoms of Encephalitis**

Slide 7-29   **Differential Field Diagnosis**
▸ Assessment of cranial infections is similar to that of a stroke. Assess the severity and manage the life threats.
▸ Dehydration from prolonged infection will produce weak, thready radial pulses. Complete a thorough neurological exam.
▸ Management is supportive. Hyperventilation at 20 per minute may be indicated. Avoid dextrose solutions to prevent cerebral edema.
▸ Treat dehydration with 20 cc/kg of isotonic crystalloid. Observe for fluid overload as it will increase ICP. Transport responsive and intubated patient semi-Fowler's position so gravity will help control ICP. Administer antibiotics.

Slide 7-30   **Differential Field Diagnosis**
▸ Remarkable facial findings

Slide 7-31   **Differential Field Diagnosis**
▸ There are two areas of insult in hemorrhagic stroke.
— One at the site of arterial rupture. This forms a hematoma. The hematoma grows and presses on the brain tissue causing ischemia to another area.
— Hypertension weakens cerebral arteries leaving them at risk for rupture.
▸ Smoking, sickle cell anemia are often contributing factors.
▸ Emotional or physical stress can be a precipitating factor.
▸ Accompanied with sudden onset and severe headache with rapid deterioration in mentation.

Slide 7-32   **Causes of Occlusive Stroke**
▸ Occlusive strokes cause blockage in arteries. This insult affects motor, sensory, and speech areas versus significant mental status changes.

▸ The signs and symptoms worsen progressively, but can often stabilize in 24–72 hours (80–85%).

▸ Often present with nausea, vomiting, hemiplegia, hemiparesis, aphasia, and dysphasia.

▸ Thrombotic—is a clot in an artery. This occlusion develops gradually because ischemia is present long before total blockage. Generally occurs at rest.

— Anti-coagulants, antiplatelets can cause thrombosis formation. Often a history of angina, atrial fibrillation.

— Pupils are generally dilated on the affected side and tend to gaze away from the affected side.

▸ Embolic incidents generally occur in the carotid artery. This is why checking for bruits prior to carotid massage can help to avoid strokes.

— Generally numbness opposite the lesion.

— Vertigo, diplopia, hemiparesis are common symptoms.

Slide 7-33   **Causes of Occlusive Stroke**

Slide 7-34   **Differential Field Diagnosis—Transient Ischemic Attack (TIA)**

Slide 7-35   **Differential Field Abnormalities of Motor Function**

▸ An abnormality in motor function is related to structural and metabolic imbalances.

▸ Metabolic imbalances can be related to thiamine deficiency.

▸ Many times the motor dysfunction is related to the intracranial pressure.

Slide 7-36   **Differential Field Diagnosis—Bizarre Behavior**

▸ A patient that is displaying bizarre behavior may have any of the following problems: stroke, cranial infection, brain tumor, hypoglycemia, alkalosis, thiamine deficiency.

▸ Lethargy and decreased LOC may be caused by diabetic emergency, acidosis, hyperthyroidism.

▸ Hyperexcitability may be caused from alkalosis and hyperthyroidism.

Slide 7-37   **Seizures**

Slide 7-38   **Differential Field Diagnosis—Seizure**

▸ Seizures and seizure disorders are among the oldest recorded diseases.

▸ It is a recurrent disorder of cerebral function with a rapid onset that is characterized by brief attacks of consciousness alteration, motor activity, sensory phenomena, or inappropriate behavior caused by abnormal discharge of cerebral neurons.

▸ To this day, seizures are poorly understood by the medical community.

Slide 7-39   **Differential Field Diagnosis—Seizure**

Slide 7-40   **Differential Field Diagnosis—Seizure**

Slide 7-41   **Important to Note**

Slide 7-42   **Important to Note**
- ▶ Examine the patient and surroundings for these medications.

Slide 7-43   **Differential Field Diagnosis of Seizures**

Slide 7-44   **Assessment and Management Priorities**

Slide 7-45   **Differential Field Diagnosis—Seizure**
- ▶ There is a relatively new classification system to the terminology of seizures. The two main classes of seizures are generalized seizures and partial seizures. Each of these is subdivided into additional classes and is based on whether the patient loses consciousness or not.
- ▶ Generalized seizures used to be called grand mal, petit mal, minor motor, etc. Bilaterally symmetrical, involving both hemispheres. Uncontrolled neural activity with loss of consciousness. The subcategories may include absence seizure (pediatric) and the tonic-clonic seizure
  - — Absence seizures: children and adolescents with sudden onset of loss of awareness; may look as though they have a blank stare with
    - ▪ amnesia of the event which ends quickly
  - — Tonic-clonic: dramatic, rapid loss of consciousness which may be accompanied by a loud cry. Tonic spasms will last 10–30 seconds then
    - ▪ clonic (contraction and relaxation) activity will begin symmetrically and may last 3–5 minutes—as long as 30 minutes.
    - ▪ a postical phase may last for hours to days and may mimic stroke in the early phase.
- ▶ Partial seizures used to be called focal motor seizures, Jacksonian seizures, temporal lobe seizures, and psychomotor seizures. They involve neurons from only one hemisphere and do not include loss of consciousness.
  - — Simple partial can include motor, sensory, and autonomic signs but no change in consciousness. Little or no postical phase.
  - — Complex partial and episodic changes in behavior— looks like a psychiatric emergency. Usually begins with an aura and includes minor muscle tremors

Slide 7-46   **Generalized Seizure**
- ▶ Involves both cerebral hemispheres. Tonic movement lasts 15–20 seconds and exhibits motor tension and tetany. Clonic movement lasts several minutes with spasms of rigidity and relaxation.
- ▶ Hypoxia and biting the tongue are risks.
- ▶ These seizures utilize 250 times the ATP energy and can cause hypoglycemia.
- ▶ Incontinence and a high-pitched cry is often present.

Slide 7-47   **Partial Seizures**
- ▶ Simple partial: Patients experience vertigo and localized contractions, for example, finger only.

	SLIDE NO.	SLIDE TITLE/NOTES

► Complex partial: aura often present.
  — Presentation appears "under the influence."
  — Repetitive movements like lip smacking, inability to concentrate and follow directions or answer questions, unconscious walking.

Slide 7-48 **Case Study 1**
► Paraphrase the information on the slide, then ask the question at the bottom. Please wait and discuss potential answers prior to moving on.
► Concerns are access in and out, multiple age-related complaints, communication issues, additional resources for support for family, awareness of unintentional aggressiveness.
► Possible causes: CNS dysfunction related to trauma, endocrine emergencies, respiratory or cardiovascular disease, renal crisis

Slide 7-49 **Scene Size-up/BSI**
► Once safety concerns are eliminated, focus on what you can hear, smell, and see.
  — Notice body positioning: flexion/decorticate, extension/decerebrate; stillness can be related to cardiac origins; erratic movements can be related to hepatic or hyperthyroid issues.
  — Tripod positioning indicates respiratory distress.
  — Facial affect of fear and anxiety may indicate severity.
  — Facial drooping indicates stroke, seizure.
► Dystonic movements of twitching and twisting are related to medications.
► Odors may indicate adverse living conditions; DKA with acetone, fruity odors, musty breath odor indicates liver dysfunction, incontinence loss of CNS function.
► Assistive devices of walkers, wheelchairs, syringes, glucometers, prosthetic devices, oxygen tubing can indicate chronic decreased cardiac output and decreased perfusion.

Slide 7-50 **Case Study 1: Scene Size-up/BSI**
► Patient is a cigarette smoker, taking drugs for high cholesterol, and hypertension medications. Patient appears ill and unstable with mentation compromise.
► Possible etiologies: respiratory, endocrine, and cardiovascular
► Airway and breathing are immediate concerns.
► Ask the question on the slide and discuss prior to moving on to the next slide.

Slide 7-51 **Case Study 1: Initial Impression**
► Answers to previous slide's question
► Ask the participants what needs to be done next and discuss prior to moving on to the next slide.

Slide 7-52 **Case Study 1: Initial Assessment**
► Initial assessment determines initial management.
► Airway concerns for stroke are impaired swallowing and for seizure, vomit and aspiration.

▶ Circulation issues from tachycardia/bradycardia and irregularity indicate potential for decreased cardiac output and decreased cerebral perfusion.

▶ Cool skin indicates cardiac etiology and compensatory shock. Hot skin indicates infection, sepsis, pneumonia, meningitis.

▶ AVPU and positioning indicate high brainstem injury. AVPU is the stimulus given to a patient and Glasgow Coma score is the response.

▶ Pupil evaluation checks third cranial nerve. In a conscious patient, pronator drift helps to evaluate neurological status.

▶ Aphasia is difficulty speaking and alters ability to assess history.

▶ Ask the question on the slide and discuss prior to moving on to the next slide.

Slide 7-53 **Case Study 1: Initial Management Considerations**

▶ Patient is unstable and has a potential life threat. Suctioning to remove secretions/gurgling respirations. Possible etiologies are TIA, hemorrhagic or occlusive stroke, seizure, hypo/hyperglycemia, head injury from recent trauma, intracranial tumor, increased ICP.

▶ Since this patient has a low level of consciousness, protection of the airway is key. Organization of patient care should include early intubation if available. A bridge device for securing the airway may be used according to protocol. Establish an IV with crystalloid at a keep open rate.

▶ Ask and discuss the two questions at the bottom of the slide prior to moving on to the next slide. Facilitate discussion with the group with positive feedback.

Slide 7-54 **Impressions**

▶ Answers to previous slide's questions

▶ Ask the next question and facilitate discussion.

Slide 7-55 **Case Study 1: SAMPLE History**

▶ Assess medication noncompliance, toxicity, and reactions to new medications.

▶ Last oral intake can reveal hydration and nutritional status, alcohol intoxication, and diabetic concerns.

▶ Events preceding can reveal recent head trauma and recent illness related to fever, headache, and stiff neck.

Slide 7-56 **Case Study 1: Focused History—OPQRST**

Slide 7-57 **Case Study 1: Focused Assessment—Vital Signs**

▶ Increased BP may indicate stroke, toxicity, hyperthyroidism, increased ICP.

▶ Bradycardia may indicate respiratory failure, increased ICP.

Slide 7-58 **Adjuncts and Interventions**

▶ The use of rapid sequence intubation using pharmacological agents may be needed to control the airway for the unconscious patient.

▶ Remember that RSI is not a rapid procedure.
▶ Aggressive hyperventilation in patients with suspected increased ICP is contraindicated.
— Excessive hyperventilation causes rapid removal of CO_2 and increases cerebral edema and decreases cerebral perfusion related to vasoconstriction.
— Hyperventilation at 15–20/minute is indicated for patients with
▪ unilateral or bilateral dilated pupils
▪ asymmetric pupil reactivity
▪ nonpurposeful posturing (flexion/extension)
▶ End tidal CO_2 recommendation is 25–30 mmHg.

Slide 7-59   **Case Study 1: Diagnostic Findings**
▶ Using diagnostic findings can lead to determining probable causes.
▶ Patient remains unstable and potential life threat.
▶ Ask the question on the slide and facilitate discussion prior to moving on. Ask additional questions related to the participants' answers, attempting to identify how to rule in or rule out the differential diagnoses.

Slide 7-60   **Case Study 1: Differential Field Diagnosis**
▶ The history many times can lead a person to what may be causing the problem.
▶ A patient that is displaying bizarre behavior may have any of the following problems: stroke, cranial infection, brain tumor, hypoglycemia, alkalosis, thiamine deficiency.

Slide 7-61   **Case Study 1: Management of Stroke**
▶ Oxygen to prevent hypercarbia, hypoxia, and acidosis.
▶ Rapid transport to appropriate facility for CT, thrombolytics, and surgery. IV of 0.9% NS. D_5W and D_{50} are contraindicated for stroke as they can increase edema as sugar metabolizes and forces hypo-osmolar fluid shifts from vessels to brain tissue.

Slide 7-62   **Case Study 1: Ongoing Assessment**
▶ Determines changes in the patient's condition.
▶ Reassess initial assessment, vital signs, focused physical exam, and effectiveness of interventions.
▶ Recent research indicates the brain may need hypertension medications during stroke. Check with medical direction with regard to treating with beta blockers.

Slide 7-63   **Case Study 2**
▶ Seizure activity increases membrane permeability to sodium and potassium increasing neurons to depolarize and create electrical charges that are abnormal. Not all seizure patients lose consciousness.
▶ Patient may be awake (functioning cerebral cortex), but not aware (decreased functioning of RAS).
▶ Initial impression: potential life threat and unstable

Slide 7-64   **Case Study 2: Scene Size-up/BSI**
▶ Bring all equipment to the patient.
▶ May need additional resources for crowd control and movement of patient.

Slide 7-65   **Case Study 2: Initial Assessment**
▶ Patient is unstable. Immediate concerns are safety and airway.
▶ Crowd control will require additional resources. Obtaining a focused history and physical exam are essential in determining the underlying causes.
▶ Underlying possibilities are endocrine emergency, recent head trauma, overdose, medication toxicity, environmental emergency, intracranial infection, etc.

Slide 7-66   **Case Study 2: Focused History**
▶ Assess for associated complaints such as aspiration, brain ischemia, and fractures.
▶ Onset and duration indicate severity.
▶ Attempt to obtain specific description of seizure type movement to assess severity and type of seizure.

Slide 7-67   **Case Study 2: Focused History**
Ask: *What is your impression after obtaining history?*
▶ Exacerbation of seizure history
— Sudden discontinuance of dilantin may exacerbate seizure activity.
— Dilantin inhibits seizure activity by altering sodium movement across cell membranes in the motor cortex.
▶ Evaluate for electrolyte imbalances.

Slide 7-68   **Case Study 2: Physical Exam and Vital Signs**

Slide 7-69   **Case Study 2: Management**
▶ Oxygenate and ventilate as appropriate. The nasopharyngeal airway might be ideal in this situation.
▶ Initiate IV therapy with isotonic crystalloid, avoid dextrose solutions.
▶ Administer benzodiazapines to stop seizure. Valium is antianxiety medication to inhibit afferent pathways to relax and stop seizure.
— Consider side effect of respiratory depression after administration.
— Can administer rectally if unable to initiate IV.

Slide 7-70   **Case Study 3: Presentation**
▶ Paraphrase the information, then ask and discuss the questions at the bottom prior to moving on to the next slide. Provide positive reinforcement.
▶ The Emergent, Urgent, Non-Urgent categories are relatively standard triage criteria in EDs.

Slide 7-71   **Case Study 3**
▶ Answers the questions from the previous slide.
▶ Ask the next question and allow discussion.

SLIDE NO.	SLIDE TITLE/NOTES
Slide 7-72	**Case Study 3: Initial Impression** ▶ Review the information and read the questions and discuss.
Slide 7-73	**Case Study 3: Initial Impression Discussion**
Slide 7-74	**Case Study 3: Vital Signs and Diagnostics** ▶ Review the normal range of glucose levels with the group and point out the fever and quiet tachypnea.
Slide 7-75	**Case Study 3: Focused History and Exam** ▶ Review this information with emphasis on the events prior to admission.
Slide 7-76	**Case Study 3: Focused History and Exam** ▶ Review the history with the participants—point out the quote from the parents about "aggressive doses" of antipyretics and the headache. ▶ Begin to ask about impression and differentials. How are differentials determined?
Slide 7-77	**Case Study 3: Focused Exam** ▶ This slide guides the participants towards some sort of infection but—with something else? ▶ Why the nystagmus, twitching, high blood sugar, low potassium, metabolic acidosis with quiet tachypnea?
Slide 7-78	**Case Study 3** ▶ Should be at least a partial list of differentials from the previous slide's question.
Slide 7-79	**Additional Information** ▶ This slide should point the participants to a HUGE dose of aspirin.
Slide 7-80	**Additional Information** ▶ Salicylate toxicity signs and symptoms ▶ Review and remind participants of the patient's presentation.
Slide 7-81	**Salicylate Overdose Treatment** ▶ Treatment overview for this malady
Slide 7-82	**Summary**

SLIDE NO.   **SLIDE TITLE/NOTES**

Slide 8-1   **Acute Abdominal Pain**
- ▶ Focus on the overview of the lecture. Limited epidemiology is offered for interest in the notes below.
  - — The acute abdomen accounts for 5% of ER visits and makes up approximately 1/3 of the surgical problems seen.
  - — Of the patients who present with acute abdominal pain, 15–30% will require surgery. This percentage is even higher in the elderly.
  - — This lecture will focus on identifying the sick vs. not sick, the affected system, and the potential life threats.

Slide 8-2   **Acute Abdomen**
Briefly summarize the process.

Slide 8-3   **Experiences and Knowledge**
- ▶ To come up with a differential diagnosis, you will need to connect the patient presentation to the disease process using the factors identified.
- ▶ Initially, you should identify several diagnoses and work to collect information through a thorough history and physical exam to identify a final diagnosis.
- ▶ As you work through the process, you will need to evaluate the risks and benefits of performing certain exams and treatments.
- ▶ Finally you should constantly reassess the patient for changes and response to the treatments you have initiated.

Slide 8-4   **Keys to Abdominal Assessment**
- ▶ When assessing the abdomen it is essential to identify life threats. You will need to look at the patient to determine if he is critical. Often, the assessment will require you to trust your instincts because a specific cause for the problem may not be initially apparent.
- ▶ Even though non-specific pain will account for 40–60% of the cases, it is essential that history be collected as is feasible.
- ▶ Emphasize not delaying transport to obtain a diagnosis.

Slide 8-5   **Implications of Abdominal Pain**
- ▶ Knowing where the pain is located and identifying the underlying organs may assist with predicting organ involvement and identifying a diagnosis.
- ▶ If the pain is not localized, it is classified as diffuse.
- ▶ Diffuse pain or poorly localized pain felt near the midline is commonly associated with peritonitis, bowel obstruction, aortic aneurysm, gastroenteritis, and pancreatitis.

	SLIDE NO.	SLIDE TITLE/NOTES

Slide 8-6 **Anatomy—Abdominal Structures**

▶ Allow participants to read the slide as you point out the following information.

— Solid organs tend to present with a constant pain.

— Hollow organs for the most part have the ability to contract or carry out peristalsis. Therefore, hollow organ pain is more commonly associated with crampy or colicky pain.

Slide 8-7 **Anatomy—Abdominal Structures**

▶ The peritoneum is the serous membrane that lines the abdominopelvic cavity. The parietal peritoneum covers the outer wall. The visceral peritoneum covers the internal organs.

▶ The peritoneum divides the abdomen vertically into the peritoneal space and the retroperitoneal space.

▶ Organs such as the kidneys, ureters, and aorta are located in the retroperitoneal space. The pancreas shares both spaces. That is why organs in the retroperitoneal space often present with back pain as opposed to anterior abdominal pain.

▶ The mesentery is a double sheet of peritoneum that supports the intestines and contains the blood vessels that supply the intestines.

▶ The skeletal structures include the vertebral column and musculature, diaphragm, and muscles of the abdominal wall.

Slide 8-8 **Pain Producing Mechanisms**

▶ Distension: Pain associated with distension is usually dependent on how rapidly the distention occurs. Rapid distention causes pain, while slow distention usually does not cause pain.

▶ Traction: Causes pain from the tension or stretching of the tissue. It is usually caused by adhesions, distention of the common bile duct, or forceful peristalsis resulting from intestinal obstruction.

▶ Edema (or vascular congestion): Can stimulate the contraction of hollow organs causing colicky or crampy pain. The edema from inflammation can also cause painful stretching.

Slide 8-9 **Pain Producing Mechanisms**

▶ Obstruction of blood vessels causes ischemic pain. Bowel obstructions stimulate pain receptors due to distention.

▶ Ischemic pain from blood vessel occlusion is steady and severe. It increases over time. Severe pain out of proportion to the findings may be ischemia pain of the mesentery.

▶ Inflammation can cause pain due to the edema and/or the chemicals released as part of the inflammatory response.

▶ Chemical irritation resulting from the inflammatory response releases histamine, bradykinin, and serotonin which stimulate nerve endings causing pain.

▶ Obstructive pain associated with ischemia increases in severity over time. The pain may seem out of proportion to the patient presentation. If so, consider immediate transport.

Slide 8-10   **Visceral Pain**

▶ Abdominal pain has multiple origins: visceral, parietal, referred, and extra-abdominal causes. Discuss and contrast the origins of abdominal pain.

▶ Visceral pain arises from the abdominal organs and is usually located in the mid-epigastric or umbilical regions near the midline of the body.

▶ It is often diffuse, vague, poorly localized because the nerve endings within the abdominal organs are sparse and multi-segmented. The pain is usually generated by stretch receptors. The nerve fibers enter the cord at several levels bilaterally so the patients may be unable to discriminate the exact location; thus the pain is perceived as diffuse.

▶ Solid organs produce a dull, constant pain. Hollow organs produce a crampy, colicky pain that is intermittent.

▶ Visceral pain may evolve into parietal pain as in the case of appendicitis.

Slide 8-11   **Parietal Pain**

▶ Parietal or somatic pain comes from the parietal peritoneum and is usually localized and intense.

▶ The nerve fibers from the parietal peritoneum travel with associated peripheral nerves of the spinal cord. The sensation of pain frequently corresponds to skin dermatomes at the T6 and L1 level. Patients can localize the pain because the pain sensation is transmitted through specific nerve fibers on the same side and at the same dermatome level as the site of the pain. Therefore, the pain tends to be unilateral.

▶ The pain is usually sharp, discrete, constant, and localized.

▶ Patients often prefer the fetal position. If you find them supine, they will often lay with their knees drawn up. This relaxes the parietal peritoneum and helps reduce the pain. Any type of movement or activity that moves the peritoneum will increase the pain. Coughing, taking a deep breath, laying flat with the legs extended, palpation, and sudden movement all increase the pain.

▶ Parietal pain frequently occurs after visceral pain, so obtaining a history describing any change in the pain is important.

Slide 8-12   **Areas of Referred Pain**

▶ This slide and the next slide (8-13) review the anterior and posterior areas of referred pain. Review the locations.
— Referred pain results from misinterpretation of sensory input by the brain.
— Ovary/fallopian tube cause referred pain due to capsule's rupturing. The release of chemicals cause irritation resulting in inflammation to the peritoneal lining, diaphragm, and phrenic nerves. This results in referred pain to either side of the neck or shoulders.
— The spleen lies near the diaphragm and left phrenic nerve. This causes referred pain to the left neck and shoulder.

— The liver lies beneath the diaphragm on the right. Inflammation and disease of the liver can result in referred pain along the phrenic nerve to the right neck and shoulder.

— The heart and lungs lie superior to the diaphragm so epigastric pain is common. The stimulation of the vagal nerve may cause associated nausea and vomiting.

— Appendicitis initially presents as visceral, poorly localized pain that may be peri-umbilical or epigastric.

— Diverticulitis presents similar to appendicitis and often causes the same type of poorly localized pain in the epigastric/umbilical area.

— Kidney stone pain is usually crampy or colicky and follows the ureter from the flank to the groin.

Slide 8-13   Areas of Referred Pain

▶ Review the locations of referred pain. Emphasize the importance of referred pain and the ability to predict organ involvement.

— Cholecystitis or gallbladder pain will be referred to the right scapula or between the scapulae

— The pancreas is located in the peritoneal and retroperitoneal space. It sits beneath the stomach and projects into the curve of the duodenum and the spleen. Since it is partially retroperitoneal, pain may be in the mid back.

— The abdominal aorta is a retroperitoneal structure. So pain from a tear in the aorta may produce visceral pain in the lumbosacral area with radiation to the anterior abdomen and legs.

— Bladder pain, because of its location, may be associated with low back pain.

— Pain associated with an AMI may refer to the arm, neck, jaw, or upper torso. This is because the visceral nerve fibers that supply the thoracic organs enter the spinal cord in the lower cervical and upper thoracic regions as do the parietal nerves fibers, once again making it difficult for the brain to localize the pain.

▶ Referred pain may be due to intra-abdominal or extra-abdominal causes.

Slide 8-14   Extra-Abdominal Causes of Pain

▶ Review the chart.

— An AMI may create diffuse abdominal pain and indigestion.

— Pneumonia may cause diffuse abdominal pain without local tenderness. Cough and fever may be present.

— In diabetic patients, elevated potassium may cause a squeezing sensation (like girdling) from the cramping of the smooth muscles.

— Drug withdrawal may present with severe colicky pain.

— Sickle cell disease patients may complain of severe abdominal pain due to splenic infarction.

— Spinal or CNS illness can cause chronic abdominal pain. The pain is often associated with inflammation of the spinal nerve roots (e.g., shingles).

▶ Remember that abdominal pain has many causes and you must focus on the patient, the presentation, and appropriate treatment, even if the exact cause of the pain is not identified.

Slide 8-15   **What is the scene telling you?**

▶ Review slide and emphasize that as part of your initial approach, you should complete a scene size-up and look for initial clues.

Slide 8-16   **Characteristics of Blood in the Gastrointestinal Tract**

▶ Review the types of bleeding and the significance of each.
— Hematemesis is associated with an upper GI bleed.
— Hematochezia is associated with a lower GI bleed. Blood is irritating to the GI tract and increases peristalsis causing diarrhea.
— Melena is a dark, black sticky stool. You often can differentiate melena from other causes of dark stool by the presence of diarrhea. Melena is often associated with diarrhea.
— Occult bleeding may not be visible in the stool if it is less than 100 cc. Chronic occult bleeding may lead to a hemoglobin loss and decrease the oxygen-carrying capacity of the blood.

Slide 8-17   **What is the scene telling you?**

▶ Look for any indicators of problems with the abdomen.
— Equipment such as indwelling catheter may indicate bladder or kidney infections or sepsis. Home dialysis should suggest infection, electrolyte imbalance.
— Look for medical alert tags.
— Look for any medications that suggest abdominal organ involvement, such as antacids.
— Odors such as vomit, GI bleed, urine smell may indicate problems.
— Condition of the kitchen may be associated with food poisoning or improper nutrition.
— Comments of bystanders and appearance of the patient are strong clues to be investigated for problems.

Slide 8-18   **What is the patient telling you?**

▶ Review the slide and emphasize patient positioning as a major indicator to potential abdominal problems.

Slide 8-19   **Initial Impression**

▶ Emphasize these factors in determining patient condition and for setting priorities.

Slide 8-20   **Focused History**

▶ Gather a history of the chief complaint by using the SAMPLE and OPQRST format. This can be done as treatment continues, or after transport is initiated.

Slide 8-21

Factors that Affect Abdominal Pain

▶ Emphasize that these factors affect the way patients perceive their pain.

— Children and infants may not be able to localize their pain so pay close attention to behavior and history.

— The obese and elderly tolerate pain better—potentially due to the presence of chronic pain or neuropathy.

— Pre-existing conditions such as the neuropathy of diabetes, alcohol, and medications such as steroids can mask abdominal pain.

Slide 8-22

Factors that Affect Abdominal Pain (continued)

▶ Patients do not perceive pain the same, so their perception of the pain severity may make the interpretation of the pain less reliable. Watch for patterns or progression. You may want to ask the patient to compare the pain to a different or previous pain incident to determine severity.

▶ The patient's mental state may affect pain perception. Hysteria coincides with an exaggeration of the pain. Emotional pain often worsens physical pain.

Slide 8-23

Clear the Systems

▶ As you are completing the assessment, it is often useful to review or clear each of the body systems. This is often useful when evaluating abdominal pain since so many of the body systems have components contained in the abdomen.

Slide 8-24

Case Study 1: Scene Size-up

Ask: *What does the scene suggest?*

— This appears to be a safe medical scene so far.

— No need for additional resources at this time.

Ask: *What is the patient telling you?*

— The patient is lying still with his knees drawn up suggesting parietal pain.

— He is in distress and not moving—possibly serious and need for early transport should be considered.

Slide 8-25

Case Study 1: Initial Assessment

▶ Initial assessment: Look for life threats and intervene if necessary.

▶ Initial impression:

— He is in distress.

— He does not appear to have

▪ an altered LOC.

▪ respiratory failure.

▪ deteriorating signs of shock.

▪ an immediate life threat.

▶ Paraphrase this information for participants.

▶ When looking for an initial impression you can also ask:

— What may be wrong with this patient?

— What else could be wrong?

— Is this patient stable or unstable?

— What should be done next?

▶ This could be a GI bleed; ruptured bowel, appendix, or other structure; sepsis; sickle cell crisis; food poisoning; etc.

▶ Oxygen, IVs, and considering early transport may also be presented.

Slide 8-26 **Case Study 1: Focused Assessment and History**

▶ Allow participants to read the vital signs; then ask them if the vital signs support their initial impressions.

Ask: *What additional information is needed?*

▶ Acceptable responses:
— The vitals suggest a patient with hypertension, tachycardia, and tachypnea. His pulse oximetry suggests a need for oxygen.
— The vitals support the impression of distress.
— The high blood pressure and pale mucous membranes do not coincide.
— Additional information includes patient history to progress to the next slide that lists SAMPLE and OPQRST.

Slide 8-27 **Case Study 1: Focused History**

▶ Paraphrase this information for participants.

▶ Look for potential life threats and intervene if necessary.

▶ Review SAMPLE for any confirmation of their initial impressions.

S Symptoms suggests: gastrointestinal involvement

A Allergies suggests: none identified

M Medications suggest: possible GI irritation, cardiovascular considerations

P Past medical problems suggest: sickle cell disease, aortic aneurysm

L Last meal combined with symptoms suggest: food poisoning

E Events suggest: a new condition or sudden exacerbation of an existing condition

▶ Other: older black male with hypertension and nausea must be evaluated for an AMI

Ask: *What additional information needs to be obtained?*
— OPQRST and other appropriate questions.

Slide 8-28 **Case Study 1: Focused History**

▶ Paraphrase this information for participants.

▶ Look for potential life threats and intervene if necessary.

▶ Use the OPQRST to confirm the initial impression.

O Onset: The rapid onset confirms a sudden change which is an indication for early transport.

P Palliation/Provocation: The presentation confirms parietal pain.

Q Quality suggests solid organ pain. The pressure-like discomfort may suggest AMI pain. Since the pain is not crampy or colicky, the diagnoses of food poisoning or hollow organ involvement is decreased.

   R Radiation: Pain goes into the back which suggests cardiac pain, aortic pain, kidney pain, pancreatic pain.

   S Severity suggests an infarction. A severe pain indicates early transport.

   T Time: The pain has stayed constant over time which supports solid organ pain, or stretch pain from aortic involvement. Tends to eliminate food poisoning or bowel involvement.

▸ Additional information would include a physical exam and a review of systems to rule out problems.

Slide 8-29

Case Study 1: Assessing Abdominal Pain
▸ Emphasize looking for life threats.
▸ This could be a life threat.

Ask: *What are your differentials?*
— Sickle cell crisis with spleen infarction is more likely, but, pancreatic disease, aortic aneurysm, ruptured ulcer, AMI, etc. are options to discuss.

Slide 8-30

Case Study 1: Physical Exam
Review and summarize.

Slide 8-31

Case Study 1: Physical Exam
Summarize.

Slide 8-32

Case Study 1: Physical Exam
Summarize.

Slide 8-33

Case Study 1: Physical Exam
Summarize.

Slide 8-34

Case Study 1: Diagnosis Sickle Cell Crisis with Splenic Infarct
Summarize. Case complete.

Slide 8-35

Case Study 2: Scene Size-up
▸ Answers reinforced:
— This appears to be a safe medical scene so far.
— No need for additional resources as yet.
— Recent dialysis, dizziness, anticoagulant use are concerns.
— Concern about hepatitis due to dialysis history should also be considered.

Slide 8-36

Case Study 2: Initial Assessment
▸ Guide participants to look for life threats and intervene if necessary.
▸ Paraphrase this information for participants.

Ask: *What may be wrong with this patient?*
What else could be wrong?
Is this patient stable or unstable?
What should be done next?

▶ This patient may be demonstrating early signs and symptoms of shock. Her airway is clear and her breathing is not compromised. Her mental status is adequate. Causes include dialysis, GI bleed, cardiac, syncope.

▶ Participants should consider getting the patient in a supine position, initiating oxygen, IVs, and considering early transport.

▶ History, vital signs, and physical exam should be the next steps.

Slide 8-37   **Case Study 2: Vital Signs**

▶ Question if the vital signs support initial impressions. Ask what additional information they need.

▶ Acceptable responses:

— The low blood pressure and pale mucous membranes correlate with GI bleed or anemia.

— A blood glucose of 90 for her could be significant; correlate it with her normal blood glucose.

— BP in right arm due to AV-shunt.

— Shock with GI bleed, sepsis, bleeding somewhere else, electrolyte imbalance, etc.

— The low pulse oximetry may be due to bleeding or anemia.

▶ This patient is showing early signs of shock. A tilt test is probably not indicated and may worsen her condition. The risk does not outweigh the benefit in this setting. If the participants opt for a tilt test, the patient would become dizzy as soon as they tried to help her sit up or stand. Allow participants to read the vital signs.

Slide 8-38   **Tilt-test**

▶ Review the slide. Point out that as in the scenario, if the patient becomes dizzy or loses consciousness, the test is positive and should be stopped.

Slide 8-39   **Case Study 2: Focused History**

▶ Paraphrase this information for participants.

▶ Look for potential life threats and intervene if necessary.

Ask: *Any confirmation of their initial impressions?*

Then ask: *What additional information needs to be obtained?*

S Her symptoms of feeling weak and dizzy suggest hypoperfusion or a syncopal episode which is consistent with the initial impression.

A None

M Her medications suggest a significant medical history and should contribute to additional discussion of differential diagnoses.

— Nitroglycerin for occasional angina suggests a cardiovascular problem.

— Tenormin is a beta 1 adrenergic blocking agent and is used for its antianginal effects and antihypertensive effects. Tenormin may also prevent the heart from increasing the rate in response to a hypotensive state. Tenormin is also associated with hypotension when given after dialysis.

— Potassium and lasix suggest a possible fluid and electrolyte imbalance.

— Erythropoietin is administered to renal failure patients because the kidney is no longer able to synthesize erythropoietin. Erythropoietin stimulates the production of red blood cells from the bone marrow. Without erythropoietin anemia results, which could contribute to her dizziness.

— Insulin indicates she is a diabetic and needs to be evaluated for her blood sugar as hypoglycemia may be a problem as well.

P Receives dialysis 2 times per week and is a diabetic, which support hypoglycemia and fluid and electrolyte imbalance. She is on anticoagulants so occult bleeding may be a problem as well.

L Ate a light lunch 2 hours ago—her sugar should still be evaluated.

E Supports possible hypovolemia and or electrolyte imbalance. The time suggests a new problem or sudden change of an old problem.

Slide 8-40

Case Study 2: Focused History
▶ Paraphrase this information for paticipants.
▶ Look for potential life threats and intervene if necessary.

Ask: *Any confirmation of your initial impressions?*
▶ Discuss the length of time she has had jelly stools and the implication.

O Indicates a recent change, or an inability to compensate.

P Exercise worsens the condition. Being still and sitting eases the condition, which reinforces hypoperfusion or a cardiac condition.

Q Denies pain.

R Denies pain.

S No complaint of pain.

T 20 minutes ago.

▶ Other: Since she is a diabetic and dialysis patient, she may have neuropathy and may not sense pain well.

Slide 8-41

Case Study 2: Focused History
▶ Neurological—The Cincinnati Stroke Test was indicated since she has several risk factors for a stroke and suffered a possible syncopal episode. Absence of neurological deficits tends to rule out stroke, but a TIA is still a possibility.
▶ Respiratory—Since she is not demonstrating any respiratory problems, the respiratory system involvement is not likely.

Slide 8-42 **Case Study 2: Focused Assessment**
▶ Her diabetic history, sex, and age may contribute to a non-classic presentation, so AMI should be considered, but aspirin and nitro are probably not indicated due to her history of heparin and hypotension.

Slide 8-43 **Case Study 2: Focused Assessment**
▶ Gastrointestinal—No, due to heparin use with dialysis, she could have occult blood loss.
▶ Renal—Since she was dialyzed today, fluid and electrolyte imbalances are possible.

Slide 8-44 **Case Study 2: Focused Assessment**
▶ Vascular—She may not compensate well to changes in pressure due to Tenormin. GI bleed is highly likely, but other causes of hypovolemia cannot be ruled out. Sepsis should also be a consideration.
▶ Consider her normal blood sugar. Many diabetics maintain a higher blood sugar as normal, so hypoglycemia may be a problem even though the readings are within the normal range.

Slide 8-45 **Case Study 2: Field Impression and Differential Diagnosis**
Review and summarize.

Slide 8-46 **Case Study 2: Gastrointestinal Bleeding**
Summarize.

Slide 8-47 **Case Study 2: Treatment of Gastrointestinal Bleeding**
Review the treatment. End of Case Study 2.

Slide 8-48 **Case Study 3: Scene Size-up**
▶ Paraphrase the information on the slide. Then ask . . .

Ask: *What does the scene suggest?*
What does the patient presentation suggest?
— This appears to be a safe medical scene so far.
— No need for additional resources as yet. Syncope and early signs of shock are a concern.

Slide 8-49 **Case Study 3: Focused History**
▶ Paraphrase this information for participants.

Ask: *What is your initial impression?*
What should be done next?
▶ Acceptable answers:
— This patient's vital signs are within normal limits.
— This could be a GI bleed.
— This could be the flu.
— She may have an ectopic pregnancy, ovarian cyst.
— She has not eaten and her blood sugar should be checked.
▶ Factors to consider:
— Tubal ligation puts her at greater risk for ectopic pregnancy.
— Since she is a marathon bicyclist, her vital signs may suggest a problem because her normal pulse is 50–54.

	SLIDE NO.	SLIDE TITLE/NOTES

Slide 8-50   **Case Study 3: Focused History**

▸ Paraphrase this information for participants.

Ask: *Does this information change or support your initial*
impression?
What else could be wrong?

▸ Acceptable answers:
 — The patient is showing early signs and symptoms of
  shock.
 — The focused history supports the previous impressions.

▸ Factors to consider:
 — Cramping indicates a hollow structure or organ
  involvement.
 — Lower abdominal pain in women must include evalua-
  tion for reproductive system diseases and problems.
 — Dizziness on standing indicates possibility of shock
  from hypovolemia.
 — LLQ cramps indicate appendix, ovary, or fallopian tube.

Slide 8-51   **Case Study 3: Focused History**

▸ Paraphrase this information for participants.

Ask: *Does the information confirm or eliminate a diagnosis?*

▸ Acceptable answers:
 — This patient is showing signs and symptoms of shock,
  and is able to compensate as long as she is flat, which
  indicates a need for early transport.
 — A GI bleed is less likely.
 — The flu is still a possibility.
 — She may have an ectopic pregnancy, ovarian cyst.

▸ Factors to consider:
 — Dizziness on standing indicates possibility of shock
  from hypovolemia.
 — LLQ cramps indicate appendix, ovary, or fallopian tube.
 — Tubal ligations have a high correlation to ectopic
  pregnancies.
 — Late period and sexually active point in the direction of
  possible pregnancy.

Slide 8-52   **Case Study 3: Follow-up**

▸ Review treatment.
 — Rapid transport is indicated.
 — Fluid replacement has improved her heart rate and was
  appropriate.

▸ When ovary/fallopian tubes rupture, they cause referred
 pain due to capsules rupturing and the chemical irritation
 from inflammation on the peritoneal lining, diaphragm, and
 phrenic nerves. This results in referred pain to either side of
 the neck or shoulders.

Slide 8-53   **Case Study 3: Follow-up**

Review. End of Case Study 3.

Slide 8-54   **Important to Note**

Remind participants that even though this lecture focused on identifying individual causes of acute abdominal pain, it is still essential to identify life threats and transport. They should not waste valuable time obtaining an in-depth field assessment on a critical or potentially critical patient.

Slide 8-55   **Summary**

Ask for questions and summarize.

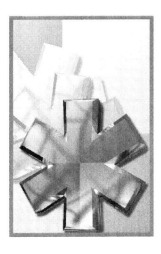

III. CASE SCENARIOS FOR PROVIDER AND REFRESHER COURSES

⊞ ASSESSMENT OF THE MEDICAL PATIENT

▶ ASSESSMENT OF THE MEDICAL PATIENT: CASE 1

Requirements: One instructor and one patient for every five participants

Prerequisite: Read Chapter 1, "Assessment of the Medical Patient" and Chapter 11, "Syncope."

Equipment: One table and chair for the patient to use; jump kit with oxygen supplies (NC, NRM, aerosol mask, PPV device, intubation equipment), stethoscope, BP cuff, cardiac monitor, pulse oximeter, and medication kit with associated medications

Instructor: Your role is vital as you must act as the coordinator of the station and also interact in the scenario. Before the participant arrives at the station, please review the scenario with your patient. Spray the patient's arms with a fine mist of cool water to simulate cool, clammy skin. Utilize moulage make-up to simulate pale skin.

Patient: One male (or female) patient. As the patient, you will be required to play the role of a 62-year-old male who has experienced a syncopal episode. You will be awake and alert. Please read the scenario to familiarize yourself with the information.

Instructions

Hi, my name is _____ , and I will be the examiner for this station. This is a hands-on patient assessment station. You will be given information concerning a patient experiencing a medical crisis. You will have all the necessary equipment you need to manage the patient in this station. Please look over the equipment before we go any further. You will be provided with pertinent information only when you ask the appropriate question. For any hands-on procedure, such as auscultation of a blood pressure or breath sounds or taking a pulse, select the appropriate equipment needed (if any) and use the equipment in the manner that it would be used on a patient. I will then give you the relevant clinical data. For example, you must select, place, and begin inflation of the BP cuff before the blood pressure is given to you. I will not answer questions in place of the patient. Therefore, it is imperative that you interact with

your patient. Please verbalize to me any signs or symptoms that you find so that I will know you are cognizant of the patient and the patient's clinical appearance.

Scenario

It is a warm humid afternoon in August. Advise the participant that she is responding to a call for a 62-year-old male who stood up to get refreshments and experienced what appears to be syncopal episode. The patient was watching his grandson's little league game. If the participant is a nurse or in-hospital provider, the scenario can be modified to the medical environment—such as a patient in the ER waiting room collapsed while standing and is being escorted to triage. The participant should use the assessment taught in this course.

Initial Impression: 62-year-old male (or female) sitting in a lawn chair with legs elevated on a cooler. The patient is positioned at the baseball field sideline.

Scene Size-up/General Impression: Local police department escorts you to the patient. Crowd control is managed and the scene is safe for entry and exit. No injury is apparent on brief visual exam. Family members surround patient and are helpful with the history of events.

Initial Assessment:
Mental Status—AVPU: A&O × 3. Patient is able to answer questions appropriately.

Airway—Clear and patent, no evidence of injury, no C-spine precautions deemed necessary

Breathing—Unlabored, equal rise of chest bilaterally, regular pattern; lungs clear

Circulation—Weak, rapid, thready radial pulse. No external bleeding. Skin is cool, pale, and moist. Pupils PERRL. Capillary refill <2 seconds. Patient can move all four extremities with equal strength. Distal pulses regular and weak.

Status after Initial Assessment: Not life threatening, potentially unstable

Initial Management Priorities: Oxygen at 4 lpm via nasal cannula, pulse oximetry, cardiac monitor, IV therapy

Focused History (SAMPLE):
Signs and Symptoms—Elderly patient seated with legs elevated in warm environment. Patient is A&O × 3, with pale, cool, clammy skin. Patient has experienced a syncopal episode.

Allergies—Penicillin

Medications—None prescribed. Patient does not take OTC medications, beta-blockers, nitrates, or diuretics.

Past Medical History—No palpitations, chest pain or difficulty breathing. No known cardiac or respiratory problems. The patient has never had a syncopal episode. No history of stroke or diabetes.

Last Oral Intake—Light lunch and ice tea

Events Preceding—Patient does not remember syncopal episode. He became syncopal when standing up to get refreshments.

OPQRST:

Onset—10 minutes prior to your arrival. When rising to get refreshments.

Palliation/Provocation—Sitting down with legs elevated

Quality—Transient, quickly resolved

Radiation—Not relevant

Severity—Brief loss of consciousness, did not fall to ground

Time/Duration—Approximately 10 seconds

Vital Signs:

Respirations—18, regular and equal in symmetry

Pulse—Radial 128 bpm, weak and rapid

Blood Pressure—92/68

Temperature—98.6°F (37°C)

Pulse Oximetry—97%

Blood Glucose Level—98 mg/dl

Focused Physical Exam (Focused Medical Assessment): Rapid head-to-toe is unremarkable. Skin tenting is negative. Neurological exam reveals no facial droop, slurred speech, and strong bilateral strength in all four extremities. There is no positive tilt test. No pedal edema.

Differential/Field Diagnosis: Self-limiting, transient loss of consciousness with loss of postural tone (syncopal episode). Contributing factors may be dehydration and remaining sedentary for a long period of time.

Management:

1) Nasal cannula at 4 lpm

2) IV access with 0.9% normal saline. Fluid bolus 200–500 ml.

3) Cardiac monitor—atrial fibrillation with no ectopy

4) Blood glucose level

5) Transport in recumbent position.

Detailed Physical Exam: En route to appropriate facility if time permits

Ongoing Assessment: There is no change in patient's condition during transport.

Critical Actions:

1) Secure airway and suction as necessary.

2) Assess for injury and use C-spine precautions if necessary.

3) Maintain hemodynamic stability with blood pressure between 70–100 mmHg.

4) Assess for underlying life-threatening etiology for syncopal episode.

Teaching Points

1) There are numerous causes and etiologies for syncope.

   a) Vasovagal syncope

   b) Orthostatic hypotension related to beta blockers, diuretics

   c) Sick sinus syndrome related to dizziness and confusion, heart blocks, symptomatic bradycardias, and sinus arrest dysrhythmias

   d) PSVT rhythms at a rate greater than 180 bpm

   e) Emotional crisis

   f) Pain

   g) Hypo/hyperglycemia with unusual behavior; BGL less than 50 mg/dl without signs and symptoms or BGL less than 60 mg/dl with signs and symptoms is considered hypoglycemic.

   h) Stroke related to neurological deficit, hemiparesis, and motor deficit

2) An organized approach and thorough patient history will assist in ruling out possible causes.

Evaluation

1) *Excellent:* The participant's evaluation of the patient followed set format: initial assessment, focused history (SAMPLE, OPQRST) in an efficient manner. The participant displayed a thorough knowledge of the patient's condition, performed the exam and management in an organized manner, and demonstrated an excellent overall performance.

2) *Good:* The participant's evaluation of the patient followed set format: initial assessment, focused history (SAMPLE, OPQRST) in an acceptable manner with only minor deviation. The participant displayed an above-average knowledge of the patient's condition, performed the exam and management of the patient's condition, and demonstrated an above-average performance.

3) *Fair:* The participant's evaluation of the patient deviated from the set format without causing any further injury to the patient. The participant displayed an average or basic knowledge of the patient's condition and performed an adequate exam and management of the patient's condition.

4) *Inadequate:* The participant's evaluation of the patient deviated significantly from the set format, or the participant's actions endangered the patient's life or significantly exacerbated the condition.

▶ Assessment of the Medical Patient: Case 2

Requirements: One instructor and one patient for every five participants

Prerequisites: Read Chapter 1, "Assessment of the Medical Patient" and Chapter 12, "Headache, Nausea, and Vomiting."

Equipment: One table and chair for the patient to use; jump kit with oxygen supplies (NC, NRM, aerosol mask, PPV device, intubation equipment), stethoscope, BP cuff, cardiac monitor, pulse oximeter, and medication kit with assorted medications

Instructor: Your role is vital as you must act as the coordinator of the station and also interact in the scenario. Before the participant arrives at the station, please review the scenario with your patient. Spray the patient's face and arms with a fine mist of cool water to simulate cool, clammy skin. Utilize moulage make-up to simulate pale skin.

Patient: One female patient. As the patient, you will be required to play the role of a 34-year-old female who has had nausea and vomiting for two days. You will be awake and alert. Please read the scenario to familiarize yourself with the information.

Instructions

Hi, my name is _____ , and I will be the examiner for this station. This is a hands-on patient assessment station. You will be given information concerning a patient experiencing a medical crisis. You will have all the necessary equipment you need to manage the patient in this station. Please look over the equipment before we go any further. You will be provided with pertinent information only when you ask the appropriate question. For any hands-on procedure, such as auscultation of a blood pressure or breath sounds or taking a pulse, select the appropriate equipment needed (if any) and use the equipment in the manner that it would be used on a patient. I will then give you the relevant clinical data. For example, you must select, place, and begin inflation of the BP cuff before the blood pressure is given to you. I will not answer questions in place of the patient. Therefore, it is imperative that you interact with your patient. Please verbalize to me any signs or symptoms that you find so that I will know you are cognizant of the patient and the patient's clinical appearance.

Scenario

Advise the participant that he is to evaluate a 34-year-old female who has had nausea and vomiting for two days. The patient is lying on a couch in her living room. If the participant is a nurse or in-hospital provider, the scenario can be modified to the medical environment—such as the patient is in ER Room 5. The participant should use the assessment taught in this course.

Initial Impression: 34-year-old female lying on a couch at residence. There is a bucket beside the couch with approximately 250 cc of vomit in it.

Scene Size-up/General Impression: Family members escort you to the patient. Family members do not speak English. There is easy acccss to the patient. No safety issues are noted. Patient is laying very still in lateral fetal position. No obvious signs of drug or alcohol use exist.

Initial Assessment:

Mental Status—AVPU: A&O × 3. Patient is able to answer questions appropriately.

Airway—No evidence of injury present. Airway clear and patent, no suction required.

Breathing—Unlabored, symmetrical chest rise; rate and rhythm regular; lungs clear.

Circulation—Bounding, rapid, and irregular radial pulse. No external bleeding noted. Skin is cool, pale, and moist. Pupils PERRL. Capillary refill 4 seconds. Patient can move all extremities with equal strength.

Status after Initial Assessment: Not life threatening, potentially unstable. No evidence of aspiration.

Initial Management Priorities: Oxygen at 4 lpm via nasal cannula, pulse oximetry, cardiac monitor, IV therapy

Focused History (SAMPLE):

Signs and Symptoms—Pale, cool, clammy skin; bounding, weak, irregular pulse; position of comfort lateral recumbent; no headache, stiff neck. Vomiting is not projectile.

Allergies—NKA

Medications—Birth control, OTC anti-emetic

Past Medical History—None other than vomiting last two days; no menses cycle problems; no risk of pregnancy

Last Oral Intake—Unable to eat or drink last two days. Has not eaten at a restaurant this week.

Events Preceding—Woke out of sleep this morning with nausea and vomiting. Has been vomiting for two days without relief of OTC anti-emetic.

OPQRST:

Onset—Last two days

Palliation/Provocation—Nothing makes it better. Vomiting not associated with food intake.

Quality—Cramping in abdomen prior to need for vomiting

Radiation—Not relevant

Severity—7 on a 10 scale

Time/Duration—Infrequent vomiting episodes yesterday, more frequent today

Vital Signs:

Respirations—24, regular and shallow, equal rise and fall of chest bilaterally

Pulse—Radial at 118 bpm, irregular and bounding

Blood Pressure—88/60

Temperature—101.2°F (38.8°C)

Pulse Oximetry—98%

Blood Glucose Level—80 mg/dl

Focused Physical Exam (Focused Medical Assessment): Rapid head-to-toe is unremarkable. Skin tenting present. Neurological exam reveals strong bilateral strength in all four extremities. Pulses weak in lower extremities. No pedal edema. No bruising, ascites, distention, rigidity, or pulsating masses to abdominal area. No pain on palpation, no rebound tenderness.

Differential/Field Diagnoses: Nausea and vomiting with hypotension, electrolyte imbalance, metabolic alkalosis, dehydration

Management:

1) Nasal cannula at 4 lpm

2) IV access with 0.9% normal saline. Fluid bolus of 200–500 ml.

3) Cardiac monitor—sinus tachycardia with occasional PACs at a rate of 118

4) Blood glucose level, D_{50} if hypoglycemic

5) Assessment of color, consistency, odor and amount of vomit

6) Administration of anti-emetics

   a) Compazine: 5–10 mg IM or IVP to block chemoreceptor trigger zone in vomit center of the brain (medulla)

   b) Phenergan: 10–25 mg PO or IM or IVP to compete with histamine for H1 receptor site in GI tract

7) Transport in position of comfort with reassessment of airway.

Detailed Physical Exam: En route to appropriate facility if time permits

Ongoing Assessment: There is no change in patient's condition during transport. Patient does not experience any vomiting episodes while under your care.

Critical Actions:

1) Secure airway and suction if necessary.

2) Maintain hemodynamic stability with blood pressure between 70–100 mmHg.

3) Assess for underlying life-threatening etiology for persistent nausea and vomiting.

Teaching Points

1) There are numerous causes and etiologies for persistent nausea and vomiting.

   a) Inner ear infections with diminished head movement

   b) If nausea is relieved after eating it may be related to gastritis. If nausea is increased after eating it may be associated with a peptic ulcer.

   c) If vomiting is projectile it may be associated with intracranial pressure.

   d) Straining when lifting or defecating may be associated concerns.

   e) Restlessness and blood in vomitus or stool may indicate obstructive (e.g., kidney stone) disease.

f) Duration and frequency of vomiting may precipitate dehydration.

g) Nausea and vomiting may be associated with posterior wall AMI, DKA, new medication toxicity or hypersensitivity, hypertensive crisis, migraine headache, or ovarian cyst.

2) An organized approach and thorough patient history will assist in ruling out possible causes.

Evaluation

1) *Excellent:* The participant's evaluation of the patient followed set format: initial assessment, focused history (SAMPLE, OPQRST) in an efficient manner. The participant displayed a thorough knowledge of the patient's condition, performed the exam and management in an organized manner, and demonstrated an excellent overall performance.

2) *Good:* The participant's evaluation of the patient followed set format: initial assessment, focused history (SAMPLE, OPQRST) in an acceptable manner with only minor deviation. The participant displayed an above-average knowledge of the patient's condition, performed the exam and management of the patient's condition, and demonstrated an above-average performance.

3) *Fair:* The participant's evaluation of the patient deviated from the set format without causing any further injury to the patient. The participant displayed an average or basic knowledge of the patient's condition and performed an adequate exam and management of the patient's condition.

4) *Inadequate:* The participant's evaluation of the patient deviated significantly from the set format, or the participant's actions endangered the patient's life or significantly exacerbated the condition.

⊞ AIRWAY MANAGEMENT

▶ AIRWAY MANAGEMENT: CASE 1

Requirements: One instructor and one manikin for every five participants

Prerequisites: Read Chapter 2, "Airway Management, Ventilation, and Oxygen Therapy."

Airway (Optional) Scenarios: Equipment
Standard precautions equipment: gloves, face shield, mask, etc.

1 adult airway manikin for every 5 participants with the following:
—Lubricant for manikin (according to manufacturer)
—Adult bag-valve-mask system
—Mouth-to-mask device for ventilation
—End-tidal CO_2 detector (colormetric)
—Esophageal detection device
—Capnography equipment (optional)
—Pulse oximeter and probe (optional)
—Cardiac monitor/defibrillator/pacer system (optional)
—Oxygen supplement appliances: non-rebreather mask, simple mask, etc. (optional)
—Stethoscope
—Various adult-sized oropharyngeal airways
—Various adult-sized nasopharyngeal airways
—Dual-lumen combination tube (CombiTube) with syringes and gastric tube *or* PtL device with syringes
—Laryngeal mask airway (LMA) with appropriate syringes (optional)
—Adult-sized (various) endotracheal tubes with syringes and stylets
—Scenario medication kit with various sedative and paralytic agents (optional)

Instructor: Your role is important as you act as the coordinator of the station, assembling and troubleshooting equipment, and act as the facilitator of the scenario presented. Before the participant arrives, arrange equipment, lubricate manikin, check laryngoscope, etc. Please read the scenarios to become familiar with the necessary responses. As the scenario is introduced to the participants involved, answer questions asked but do not offer more information than would be obvious in looking at a patient. NOTE: There are only 2 scenarios in this set as there is no testing in this topic.

Instructions

Hi, my name is _____ , and I will be the examiner for this station. This is a hands-on patient assessment station. You will be given information concerning a patient experiencing a medical crisis. You will have all the necessary equipment you need to manage the patient in this station. Please look over the equipment before we go any further. You will be provided with pertinent information only when you ask the appropriate question. For any hands-on procedure, such as auscultation of a blood pressure or breath sounds or taking a pulse, select the appropriate equipment needed (if any) and use the equipment in the manner that it would be used on a patient. I will then give you the relevant clinical data. For example, you must select, place, and begin inflation of the BP cuff before the blood pressure is given to you. I will not answer questions in place of the patient. Therefore, it is imperative that you interact with your patient. Please verbalize to me any signs or symptoms that you find so that I will know you are cognizant of the patient and the patient's clinical appearance.

Scenario

Advise the participant that she is responding to a local, small hospital to transport a medical patient to another facility with specialized resources. The participant should use the assessment taught in this course.

Initial Impression: 56-year-old female lying on the Emergency Department cart with eyes closed, pale, working hard to breathe, with tachypnea.

Scene Size-up/General Impression: Scene is safe. No obvious trauma noted. This patient appears to weigh approximately 150 lbs (68 kg).

Initial Assessment:

Mental Status—Responds to painful stimuli by pushing your hand away (localizes).

Airway—No secretions visible. Swallows without effort spontaneously. Air is moving.

Breathing—Respiratory effort labored with accessory muscle use and at an increased rate. Breath sounds are heard easily throughout fields without crackles.

Circulation—Skin color is pale, warm, and dry. Radial pulses palpable at 90 per minute. No verbal response. Does not follow commands. Glasgow Coma score of 7. Moves all extremities spontaneously.

Status after Initial Assessment: Unstable, potential life threat

Initial Management Priorities: NRM, cardiac monitor, pulse oximetry, IV therapy. Be prepared for BVM ventilation.

Focused History (SAMPLE):

Signs and Symptoms—The nurse at the bedside relates that this 56-year-old was admitted to their ED this A.M. (2 hours ago) with decreased level of consciousness.

Allergies—Codeine

Medications—Humulin insulin—regular and NPH; enteric coated aspirin; potassium; lasix; digitalis; nifedipine

Past Medical History—Diabetes, hypertension, heart disease

Last Oral Intake—Unknown—was found by a neighbor like this

Events Preceding—Patient lives on her own. Neighbor found her this A.M. on the couch in this state. Neighbor thought she was OK these past 2 days—not sure.

OPQRST:

Onset—Found 2 hours ago. Last seen up and about 2 days ago.

Palliation/Provocation—Patient not conversant.

Quality—Patient not conversant.

Radiation—Not applicable

Severity—Not applicable

Time/Duration—Found 2 hours ago; unknown duration. Patient's apartment seemed slightly messy—"not like her," according to neighbor.

Vital Signs:
Respirations—30, deep

Pulse—90 bpm at the radius

Blood Pressure—150/100

Temperature—101°F (38.3°C)

Pulse Oximetry—92% on room air, 95% with oxygen via non-rebreather

Blood Glucose Level—800 mg/dl on admission

Focused Physical Exam (Focused Medical Assessment): Head-to-toe exam reveals a slightly obese female with distended abdomen who is working hard to breathe. No obvious trauma, no open wounds, no obvious signs of infection. Sinus tachycardia on lead 2. ABGs in the ED show pH of 7.10, pCO_2 of 15, pO_2 of 90, HCO_3 –12 with base excess of –6.

Differential/Field Diagnosis: Diabetic ketoacidosis with low level of consciousness

Management:
1) Due to patient's low level of consciousness, definitive airway management for airway protection should be performed prior to commencing transfer.

   a) High-flow oxygen is being administered.

   b) 2 IVs should be established.

   c) All monitoring equipment applied.

   d) RSI protocol should be followed. (Participant should check potassium level if using succinylcholine.)

   e) Appropriately-sized endotracheal tube inserted, assessed for placement using two techniques, and secured at the proper depth.

   f) Participant should discuss RSI failed intubation protocols.

   NOTE: If EMT-Bs are participating in these groups, they are integral in assisting in RSI procedures. Make sure they understand their role in providing Sellick's maneuver, BVM ventilation, etc.

2) Discuss appropriate respiratory assessment during transport.

3) Continue monitoring and medication administration for assisted respiration during transport.

4) Discuss proper ventilation rate and depth occur.

Detailed Physical Exam: En route to appropriate facility as time permits

Ongoing Assessment: Continue evaluation of respiratory effort and level of consciousness

Critical Actions:

1) Recognize the potential for airway and ventilation problems during the transfer of a patient with a diminished Glasgow Coma score.

2) Proper assessment for and demonstration of the generic protocol for medication-assisted intubation techniques.

3) Management of the intubated patient with positive pressure ventilation in regards to proper monitoring techniques, continued sedation and paralytic administration, and ventilation therapy.

Teaching Points

1) For a complicated medical patient such as described in this case, an advanced level of EMS care should be provided. This advanced care should include good assessment and management skills for airway and ventilation therapy.

2) The groups should discuss alternative airway securement options if RSI is not available. They should also discuss what options the EMS crews have if the local physician performs RSI and expects them to continue sedation and paralytic administration without having appropriate protocols.

3) There are literally hundreds of variances in how to perform RSI. Each advanced EMS crew should follow their Medical Director's guidance in this procedure and understand every nuance of their protocol.

4) The pathophysiology involved in this case includes an insulin-dependent diabetic in diabetic ketoacidosis (DKA). The instructor should discuss causes of DKA, common clinical findings, and treatment. The case should create discussion on the possibility of this patient having hyperkalemia and the consequences of that within certain RSI protocols with options available (e.g., Succinylcholine should be avoided in cases with hyperkalemia.).

Evaluation *(NOTE: This is a teaching station, not a tested station.)*

1) *Excellent:* The participants evaluated and recognized the need for a more secure airway prior to transport. They worked as a team to complete the medical assessment of the patient including SAMPLE, OPQRST, and a focused exam. They assessed for complications of intubation and use of the RSI procedure; they had a back-up plan in place for the potential for failed RSI. They demonstrated good skills and discussed appropriate monitoring and ventilation technique.

2) *Good:* The group evaluated the patient using the standard medical assessment format and recognized the patient with a low level of consciousness with potential for airway compromise. They displayed an above-average knowledge of advanced airway management and alternatives for this patient's condition. They were able to perform the skills of airway management and discussed with the instructor the steps in RSI and complications.

3) *Fair:* The group evaluated the patient with some assistance from the instructor. They recognized the need for advanced airway management but had to be taught how to perform these procedures. They followed the lead of the instructor in assessing for complications of intubation and RSI. They could provide basic airway and ventilation skills with assistance in pathophysiology of this case.

4) *Inadequate:* The entire station had to be taught by the instructor. The group was unable to provide a medical assessment, unable to identify pathophysiology, and unable to appropriately manage the basics without being led by the instructor.

▶ Airway Management: Case 2

Requirements: One instructor and one manikin for every five participants

Prerequisites: Read Chapter 2, "Airway Management, Ventilation, and Oxygen Therapy."

Airway (Optional) Scenarios: Equipment
Standard precautions equipment: gloves, face shield, mask, etc.

1 adult airway manikin for every 5 participants with the following:
—Lubricant for manikin (according to manufacturer)
—Adult bag-valve-mask system
—Mouth-to-mask device for ventilation
—End-tidal CO_2 detector (colormetric)
—Esophageal detection device
—Capnography equipment (optional)
—Pulse oximeter and probe (optional)
—Cardiac monitor/defibrillator/pacer system (optional)
—Oxygen supplement appliances: non-rebreather mask, simple mask, etc. (optional)
—Stethoscope
—Various adult-sized oropharyngeal airways
—Various adult-sized nasopharyngeal airways
—Dual-lumen combination tube (CombiTube) with syringes and gastric tube *or* PtL device with syringes
—Laryngeal mask airway (LMA) with appropriate syringes (optional)
—Adult-sized (various) endotracheal tubes with syringes and stylets
—Scenario medication kit with various sedative and paralytic agents (optional)

Instructor: Your role is important as you act as the coordinator of the station, assembling and troubleshooting equipment, and act as the facilitator of the scenario presented. Before the participant arrives, arrange equipment, lubricate manikin, check laryngoscope, etc. Please read the scenarios to become familiar with the necessary responses. As the scenario is introduced to the participants involved, answer questions asked but do not offer more information than would be obvious in looking at a patient. NOTE: There are only 2 scenarios in this set as there is no testing in this topic.

Instructions

Hi, my name is _____ , and I will be the examiner for this station. This is a hands-on patient assessment station. You will be given information concerning a patient experiencing a medical crisis. You will have all the necessary equipment you need to manage the patient in this station. Please look over the equipment before we go any further. You will be provided with pertinent information only when you ask the appropriate question. For any hands-on procedure, such as auscultation of a blood pressure or breath sounds or taking a pulse, select the appropriate equipment needed (if any) and use the equipment in the manner that it would be used on a patient. I will then give you the relevant clinical data. For example, you must select, place, and begin inflation of the BP cuff before the blood pressure is given to you. I will not answer questions in place of the patient. Therefore, it is imperative that you interact with

your patient. Please verbalize to me any signs or symptoms that you find so that I will know you are cognizant of the patient and the patient's clinical appearance.

Scenario

Advise the participant that he is responding to a rural farm residence at 08:00 for an older gentleman whose wife states, "He won't wake up." If the participant is a nurse or in-hospital provider, this scenario can be modified to the medical environment—such as an elderly female drives up to the ED doors with her husband in the back seat of the car. The participant should use the assessment taught in this course.

Initial Impression: An elderly, thin male with his eyes closed; pale, no visible increased work of breathing.

Scene Size-up/General Impression: Century-old farmhouse with patient in upstairs bedroom. No scene hazards but potential for problems in getting this patient down the narrow steps. (Alternative: Patient in backseat of car—make sure car is off.) Frantic wife is present.

Initial Assessment:
Mental Status—Unresponsive to your verbal stimuli, extends to painful stimuli.

Airway—Some saliva in the mouth; intact gag reflex. Air is moving noisily.

Breathing—Slow rise and fall of the chest with breath sounds shallow only. Some loud, upper airway noise is heard.

Circulation—Radial pulses palpable at a slow rate. Skin is cool and pale.

Disability—Pupils are unequal: Right is at 6 mm, left is at 2 mm (no signs of cataracts). Extends to painful stimuli.

Status After Initial Assessment: Unstable, serious, potential life threat—needs immediate management.

Initial Management Priorities: Immediate suctioning and assisted ventilations; after heart rate increases—cardiac monitor, IV therapy.

Focused History (SAMPLE):
Signs and Symptoms—Wife unable to awaken her husband. Felt OK yesterday.

Allergies—NKA

Medications—Vitamins, otherwise no medications

Previous History—"Broken leg when he was young"—otherwise no history. Hasn't seen a doctor in 20 years.

Last Oral Intake—Last night at about 6:00 P.M. (14 hours ago)

Events Preceding—Went to bed at usual time last evening. Nothing unusual.

OPQRST:
Onset—Sometime in the night

Palliation/Provocation—Not applicable

Quality—Not applicable

Radiation—Not applicable

Severity—Not applicable

Time/Duration—Attempted to awaken him at 08:00—he usually rises at 06:00.

Vital Signs:

Respirations—6 breaths per minute, without assistance

Pulse—45 bpm prior to positive pressure ventilation (PPV)
80 bpm with PPV

Blood Pressure—180/110

Temperature—96°F (35.6°C)

Pulse Oximetry—85% on room air; 95% with PPV

Capnography—65 with spontaneous respirations; 40 with PPV

Blood Glucose Level—80 mg/dl

Focused Physical Exam (Focused Medical Assessment): Rapid head-to-toe is negative except for unequal pupils, as described earlier. No signs of trauma.

Differential/Field Diagnosis: Hemorrhagic CVA

Management:

1) Immediate airway suctioning

2) Ventilatory assistance with high-flow oxygen at a rate of 12–15 per minute

3) IV access with minimal fluid administration

4) Cardiac and respiratory monitors

5) Advanced airway management with use of sedation vs. sedation and paralytic

6) Transport to the nearest appropriate medical center for stroke

Detailed Physical Exam: En route to appropriate facility as time permits

Ongoing Assessment: There is no change in patient's condition during transport.

Critical Actions:

1) Basic and advanced airway techniques performed within the initial assessment for the basic techniques and the advanced techniques once the entire assessment and focused exam are completed.

2) Recognizing the need for rapid transport of a critically-ill patient with a time-critical medical problem.

Teaching Points

1) The assessment should point the participants towards a catastrophic, acute medical problem such as CVA. The instructor should review the differences in presentation of ischemic vs. hemorrhagic CVA. The instructor should also discuss differential diagnoses in the patient with acute loss of consciousness.

2) Since the patient postures with painful stimuli and has an intact gag reflex, providing an advanced airway may prove difficult. Use of RSI or alternative means of advanced airway management should be discussed (e.g., nasotracheal route vs. RSI; use of sedation alone vs. use of sedation and paralytics). Discuss concerns regarding the increase in intracranial pressure.

3) Discussion should include whether to quickly facilitate transfer off the scene for a patient with a time-critical problem vs. staying and providing a more advanced airway, depending upon scene-hospital proximity.

Evaluation *(NOTE: This is a teaching station, not a testing station)*

1) *Excellent:* The participants were able to complete the medical assessment thoroughly, without prompting by the instructor. They were able to provide a field impression and differentials with tactics to rule in or out causes of unconsciousness. Critical thinking skills were attuned to providing basic and advanced airway management with thoughts towards scene time and proximity to an appropriate hospital and use of alternative advanced airway techniques vs. sedation only assistance vs. full RSI protocol use.

2) *Good:* The group was able to complete the medical assessment with minimal prompting by the instructor and with some organization. They were able to provide most of the differentials for the patient with acute unconsciousness and appropriate management for each. They were able to demonstrate good basic and advanced airway techniques. They were able to participate in the discussion, led by the instructor, on use of medication-assisted intubation, complications, and contraindications.

3) *Fair:* The participants were able to provide some aspects of the medical assessment and initial management without harm to the patient. Average knowledge in advanced airway techniques available to the patient in this case was demonstrated. Instructor had to lead most of the discussion on scene time for CVA vs. advanced airway management.

4) *Inadequate:* The group was unable to assess and manage the patient with acute unconsciousness, nor able to differentiate the possible causes. Their knowledge of management techniques for airway were lacking.

⊞ HYPOPERFUSION (SHOCK)

▶ HYPOPERFUSION (SHOCK): CASE 1

Requirements: One instructor and one patient for every five participants

Prerequisites: Read Chapter 4, "Hypoperfusion (Shock)."

Equipment: One table and chair for the patient to use; jump kit with oxygen supplies (NC, NRM, aerosol mask, PPV device, intubation equipment), stethoscope, BP cuff, cardiac monitor, pulse oximeter, and medication kit with assorted medications

Instructor: Your role is vital as you must act as the coordinator of the station and also interact in the scenario. Before the participant arrives at the station, please review the scenario with your patient. For moulage, tint the patient's arms and anterior chest red to simulate erythema.

Patient: One male (or female) patient. As the patient, you will be required to play the role of a 28-year-old male suffering from difficulty in breathing and increasing signs of shock due to an anaphylactic reaction from a bee sting. You are alert and very agitated. When asked questions, you are initially able to communicate but with great difficulty. You were cutting grass when you felt a burning in your leg. Please read the scenario to familiarize yourself with the information.

Instructions

Hi, my name is _____ , and I will be the examiner for this station. This is a hands-on patient assessment station. You will be given information concerning a patient experiencing a medical crisis. You will have all the necessary equipment you need to manage the patient in this station. Please look over the equipment before we go any further. You will be provided with pertinent information only when you ask the appropriate question. For any hands-on procedure, such as auscultation of a blood pressure or breath sounds or taking a pulse, select the appropriate equipment needed (if any) and use the equipment in the manner that it would be used on a patient. I will then give you the relevant clinical data. For example, you must select, place, and begin inflation of the BP cuff before the blood pressure is given to you. I will not answer questions in place of the patient. Therefore, it is imperative that you interact with your patient. Please verbalize to me any signs or symptoms that you find so that I will know you are cognizant of the patient and the patient's clinical appearance.

Scenario

Advise the participant that she is called to a residence for difficulty in breathing. When she arrives she finds a pale, extremely diaphoretic male (or female) patient pacing up and down the driveway. If the participant is a nurse or in-hospital provider, the scenario can be modified to the medical environment—such as having the patient pull his/her car up to the front door of the ED and run to the triage desk, where the participant is sitting. The participant should use the assessment taught in this course.

Initial Impression: 28-year-old male (or female) suffering from acute difficulty in breathing.

Scene Size-up/General Impression: The scene is safe for entry and exit. There is no apparent injury on brief visual exam. The patient appears ill.

Initial Assessment:

Mental Status—Responsive and visibly agitated, alert and oriented to person, place, and time (A&O × 3)

Airway—Audible wheezes coming from patient

Breathing—Respirations 34 and shallow, breath sounds absent in the bases, wheezing in the apexes, very little air movement

Circulation—Radial pulse weak, skin cool and clammy

Disability—Moves all four extremities

Status after Initial Assessment: Serious, airway management initial concern

Initial Management Priorities: High-flow oxygen at 15 lpm via NRM, IV access, blood glucose level, cardiac monitor, position of comfort

Focused History (SAMPLE):

Signs and Symptoms—Agitated, audible airway sounds; decreased respiratory movement; weak radial pulses; cool and clammy extremities

Allergies—Milk

Medications—Patient denies any.

Past Medical History—Patient denies.

Last Oral Intake—This A.M.

Events Preceding—Patient explains that he was cutting grass and felt a burning sensation in leg.

OPQRST:

Onset—Unknown; the patient is having extreme difficulty talking.

Palliation/Provocation—Worsens when the patient is placed in a supine position

Quality—Unknown; the patient is having extreme difficulty talking.

Radiation—Unknown; the patient is having extreme difficulty talking.

Severity—If participant asks the patient if this reaction is worse than before, he will shake his head yes.

Time—Unknown; the patient is having extreme difficulty talking.

Vital Signs:

Respirations—Too fast to count, minimal chest rise and fall

Pulse—Radial pulse weak, barely palpable

Blood Pressure—98/palpation

Temperature—99.2°F (37.6°C)

Pulse Oximetry—92%

Blood Glucose Level—102 mg/dl

Focused Physical Exam (Focused Medical Assessment): Erythema to anterior chest and arms

Differential/Field Diagnosis: Distributive shock (anaphylactic reaction)

Management:

1) High-flow oxygen at 15 lpm via NRM; if insufficient respiratory movement, then PPV

2) Epinephrine 1:1,000 0.3–0.5 mg SQ

3) IV access $\times$ 1, fluid bolus to maintain 70–100 mmHg BP

4) Diphenhydramine 25 mg IVP

5) Cardiac monitor—sinus tachycardia with frequent premature ventricular contractions (PVCs)

Detailed Physical Exam: En route to receiving facility if time permits

Ongoing Assessment: Continue to monitor respirations. Position patient for comfort.

Critical Actions:

1) Secure the airway and ensure highest oxygenation at 15 lpm via NRM.

2) If unstable airway, then PPV with rapid sequence intubation (RSI).

3) Maintain aggressive treatment with fluid bolus, epinephrine, and dopamine because of patient's condition.

Teaching Points

1) There are numerous causes and etiologies of difficulty of breathing, and the focus should remain on assessment.

2) Always follow an organized approach to rule out possible causes.

3) Don't let past medical history lead you to a diagnosis preemptively.

4) Treatment priority is aggressive management to correct for cardiopulmonary collapse.

5) Explain the advantages and disadvantages of using an RSI.

Evaluation

1) *Excellent:* The participant's evaluation of the patient followed set format: initial assessment, focused history (SAMPLE, OPQRST) in an efficient manner. The participant displayed a thorough knowledge of the patient's condition, performed the exam and management in an organized manner, and demonstrated an excellent overall performance.

2) *Good:* The participant's evaluation of the patient followed set format: initial assessment, focused history (SAMPLE, OPQRST) in an acceptable manner with only minor deviation. The participant displayed an above-average knowledge of the patient's condition, performed the exam and management of the patient's condition, and demonstrated an above-average performance.

3) *Fair:* The participant's evaluation of the patient deviated from the set format without causing any further injury to the patient. The participant displayed an average or basic knowledge of the patient's condition and performed an adequate exam and management of the patient's condition.

4) *Inadequate:* The participant's evaluation of the patient deviated significantly from the set format, or the participant's actions endangered the patient's life or significantly exacerbated the condition.

▶ HYPOPERFUSION (SHOCK): CASE 2

Requirements: One instructor and one patient for every five participants

Prerequisites: Read Chapter 4, "Hypoperfusion (Shock)."

Equipment: One table and chair for the patient to use; jump kit with oxygen supplies (NC, NRM, aerosol mask, PPV device, intubation equipment), stethoscope, BP cuff, cardiac monitor, pulse oximeter, and medication kit with assorted medications

Instructor: Your role is vital as you must act as the coordinator of the station and also interact in the scenario. You will also act as the nurse who is responsible for this patient. When EMS arrives, you state that the patient has had a high fever (104.2°F/40.4°C) for approximately 12 hours that has not been relieved with Tylenol. The doctor was notified because the patient was no longer responsive, and he ordered the patient sent to the emergency department (ED) for evaluation. After that you can tell the participant that you must tend to another patient and you will no longer be available. Before the participant arrives at the station, please review the scenario with your patient.

Patient: One female (or male) patient. As the patient, you will be required to play the role of a 74-year-old female suffering from an elevated temperature. You will be responsive only to painful stimuli with purposeful movement (attempt to move away from the pain). Please read the scenario to familiarize yourself with the information.

Instructions

Hi, my name is _____ , and I will be the examiner for this station. This is a hands-on patient assessment station. You will be given information concerning a patient experiencing a medical crisis. You will have all the necessary equipment you need to manage the patient in this station. Please look over the equipment before we go any further. You will be provided with pertinent information only when you ask the appropriate question. For any hands-on procedure, such as auscultation of a blood pressure or breath sounds or taking a pulse, select the appropriate equipment needed (if any) and use the equipment in the manner that it would be used on a patient. I will then give you the relevant clinical data. For example, you must select, place, and begin inflation of the BP cuff before the blood pressure is given to you. I will not answer questions in place of the patient. Therefore, it is imperative that you interact with your patient. Please verbalize to me any signs or symptoms that you find so that I will know you are cognizant of the patient and the patient's clinical appearance.

Scenario

Advise the participant that he is responding to a call at the local nursing home for a "resident who is ill." If the participant is a nurse or in-hospital provider, the scenario can be modified to the medical environment—such as reporting to triage after a shift change where the patient is found near the triage desk slumped over in a wheelchair. The participant should use the assessment taught in this course.

Initial Impression: 74-year-old female (or male) nursing home patient lying in bed

Scene Size-up/General Impression: There is no apparent signs of injury on brief visual exam. Wheelchairs have been moved for easy access to patient.

Initial Assessment:

   Mental Status—Only responsive (purposeful movement) to painful stimuli

   Airway—Clear at this time

   Breathing—Respirations 36 and very shallow, crackles in the bases

   Circulation—Radial pulse weak and thready at 116 bpm, barely palpable, skin very warm and dry to the touch

   Disability—Painful withdrawal in all four extremities

Status after Initial Assessment: Unstable, potential life threat

Initial Management Priorities: High-flow oxygen at 15 lpm via NRM, IV access, cardiac monitor, position of comfort

Focused History (SAMPLE):

   Signs and Symptoms—Only responsive to painful stimuli, weak radial pulse, warm and dry skin, crackles in the bases of the lungs

   Allergies—On transfer sheet, penicillin, amoxicillin, vancomycin

   Medications—On transfer sheet, Humulin N, aspirin, Cardizem

   Past Medical History—On transfer sheet, IDDM and A-Fib

   Last Oral Intake—Unknown

   Events Preceding—Already stated by nurse who left the room

OPQRST:

   Onset—About 12 hours ago

   Palliation/Provocation—Unknown

   Quality—Unknown

   Radiation—Unknown

   Severity—Unknown

   Time—Unknown

Vital Signs:

   Respirations—36 and very shallow

   Pulse—Radial pulse rapid and weak at 116 bpm

   Blood Pressure—68/palpation

   Temperature—104.6°F (40.7°C)

   Pulse Oximetry—Reading error

   Blood Glucose Level—82 mg/dl

Focused Physical Exam (Focused Medical Assessment): No injury. Bruising from insulin injections noted on left upper quadrant of abdomen. Large decubitus ulcer on right thigh and buttocks.

Differential/Field Diagnosis: Distributive shock (sepsis)

Management:

1) Supplemental oxygen at 15 lpm via NRM; if respiratory failure, then PPV

2) IV access × 2, fluid bolus to maintain a systolic BP between 70–100 mmHg

3) Cardiac monitor—atrial fibrillation

4) Consider dopamine 5–10 µg/kg/min to increase pressure

5) Transport

Detailed Physical Exam: Rapid head-to-toe physical exam to identify potential for abuse, neglect, or previous injury

Ongoing Assessment: There is no change in patient's condition during transport.

Critical Actions:

1) Secure airway and ensure highest oxygenation at 15 lpm via NRM; if respiratory failure, then PPV.

2) Maintain hemodynamic stability—BP between 70–100 mmHg, no higher.

Teaching Points

1) There are numerous causes and etiologies of hypoperfusion/shock.

2) Always follow an organized approach to rule out possible causes.

3) Treatment priorities are to maintain oxygenation and hemodynamic stability.

Evaluation

1) *Excellent:* The participant's evaluation of the patient followed set format: initial assessment, focused history (SAMPLE, OPQRST) in an efficient manner. The participant displayed a thorough knowledge of the patient's condition, performed the exam and management in an organized manner, and demonstrated an excellent overall performance.

2) *Good:* The participant's evaluation of the patient followed set format: initial assessment, focused history (SAMPLE, OPQRST) in an acceptable manner with only minor deviation. The participant displayed an above-average knowledge of the patient's condition, performed the exam and management of the patient's condition, and demonstrated an above-average performance.

3) *Fair:* The participant's evaluation of the patient deviated from the set format without causing any further injury to the patient. The participant displayed an average or basic knowledge of the patient's condition and performed an adequate exam and management of the patient's condition.

4) *Inadequate:* The participant's evaluation of the patient deviated significantly from the set format, or the participant's actions endangered the patient's life or significantly exacerbated the condition.

▶ HYPOPERFUSION (SHOCK): CASE 3

Requirements: One instructor and one patient for every five participants

Prerequisites: Read Chapter 4, "Hypoperfusion (Shock)."

Equipment: One table and chair for the patient to use; jump kit with oxygen supplies (NC, NRM, aerosol mask, PPV device, intubation equipment), stethoscope, BP cuff, cardiac monitor, pulse oximeter, and medication kit with assorted medications

Instructor: Your role is vital as you must act as the coordinator of the station and also interact in the scenario. Before the participant arrives at the station, please review the scenario with your patient. Spray the patient's arms with a fine mist of cool water to simulate cool and clammy skin.

Patient: One female patient. As the patient, you will be required to play the role of a 26-year-old female complaining of difficulty breathing. Your breathing difficulty and cardiovascular collapse are caused by a massive pulmonary embolism. You will be responsive and answer all questions. Please read the scenario to familiarize yourself with all the information. You will have a fine mist of water sprayed on you to simulate cool and diaphoretic skin.

Instructions

Hi, my name is _____ , and I will be the examiner for this station. This is a hands-on patient assessment station. You will be given information concerning a patient experiencing a medical crisis. You will have all the necessary equipment you need to manage the patient in this station. Please look over the equipment before we go any further. You will be provided with pertinent information only when you ask the appropriate question. For any hands-on procedure, such as auscultation of a blood pressure or breath sounds or taking a pulse, select the appropriate equipment needed (if any) and use the equipment in the manner that it would be used on a patient. I will then give you the relevant clinical data. For example, you must select, place, and begin inflation of the BP cuff before the blood pressure is given to you. I will not answer questions in place of the patient. Therefore, it is imperative that you interact with your patient. Please verbalize to me any signs or symptoms that you find so that I will know you are cognizant of the patient and the patient's clinical appearance.

Scenario

Advise the participant that she is responding to a call for difficulty breathing at a local bus depot. If the participant is a nurse or in-hospital provider, the scenario can be modified to the medical environment—such as having a taxi driver pull up to the ED doors and ask for assistance in removing the patient. The participant should use the assessment taught in the course.

Initial Impression: 26-year-old female sitting in a chair, answering questions

Scene Size-up/General Impression: Ill female sitting on the curb next to the bus. No evidence of trauma.

Initial Assessment:

Mental Status—Responsive and alert to all commands

Airway—Clear and patent at this time

Breathing—Respirations 46 and very shallow

Circulation—Radial pulse irregular at 106 bpm, skin cool and diaphoretic

Disability—Moves all four extremities

Status after Initial Assessment: Unstable, potential life threat.

Initial Management Priorities: High-flow oxygen at 15 lpm via NRM, percuss lung sounds, cardiac monitor, IV access, position of comfort

Focused History (SAMPLE):

Signs and Symptoms—Patient sitting upright and leaning forward, shallow respirations, cool and clammy skin

Allergies—Aspirin

Medications—Birth control

Past Medical History—Patient has smoked two packs of cigarettes a day for 10 years

Last Oral Intake—A McDonald's Happy Meal about 2 hours ago, at a bus stop

Events Preceding—Patient stated she developed a sharp pain in her chest after she stood up and got off the bus. (If the participant inquires further, the bus trip was 16 hours long.)

OPQRST:

Onset—Very sudden, when I stood up.

Palliation/Provocation—Anytime I move from a sitting position, it gets worse.

Quality—It's very sharp.

Radiation—It's just in my chest.

Severity—The pain and difficulty breathing rank a 7.

Time—It's been going on for about 20 minutes.

Vital Signs:

Respirations—46 and shallow

Pulse—Radial pulse irregular at 96 bpm

Blood Pressure—84/76

Temperature—98.5°F (37.0°C)

Pulse Oximetry—91%

Focused Physical Exam (Focused Medical Assessment): Unremarkable.

Differential/Field Diagnosis: Obstructive shock (pulmonary embolism)

Management:
1) High-flow oxygen at 15 lpm via NRM

2) IV access—fluid bolus to maintain a systolic BP of 70–100 mmHg

3) Cardiac monitor—sinus tachycardia with multifocal PVCs

4) Transport

Detailed Physical Exam: En route to appropriate facility if time permits

Ongoing Assessment: Continue to monitor respiratory status. Monitor vital signs.

Critical Actions:
1) Secure the airway and ensure highest oxygenation at 15 lpm via NRM; if respiratory failure, then PPV.

2) Maintain hemodynamic stability—BP between 70–100 mmHg, no higher.

Teaching Points

1) There are numerous causes and presentations of shock.

2) Always follow an organized approach to rule out possible causes.

Evaluation

1) *Excellent:* The participant's evaluation of the patient followed set format: initial assessment, focused history (SAMPLE, OPQRST) in an efficient manner. The participant displayed a thorough knowledge of the patient's condition, performed the exam and management in an organized manner, and demonstrated an excellent overall performance.

2) *Good:* The participant's evaluation of the patient followed set format: initial assessment, focused history (SAMPLE, OPQRST) in an acceptable manner with only minor deviation. The participant displayed an above-average knowledge of the patient's condition, performed the exam and management of the patient's condition, and demonstrated an above-average performance.

3) *Fair:* The participant's evaluation of the patient deviated from the set format without causing any further injury to the patient. The participant displayed an average or basic knowledge of the patient's condition and performed an adequate exam and management of the patient's condition.

4) *Inadequate:* The participant's evaluation of the patient deviated significantly from the set format, or the participant's actions endangered the patient's life or significantly exacerbated the condition.

▶ HYPOPERFUSION (SHOCK): CASE 4

Requirements: One instructor and one patient for every five participants

Prerequisites: Read Chapter 4, "Hypoperfusion (Shock)."

Equipment: One table and chair for the patient to use; jump kit with oxygen supplies (NC, NRM, aerosol mask, PPV device, intubation equipment), stethoscope, BP cuff, cardiac monitor, pulse oximeter, and medication kit with assorted medications

Instructor: Your role is vital as you must act as the coordinator of the station and also interact in the scenario. Before the participant arrives at the station, please review the scenario with your patient. Spray the patient's arms with a fine mist of cool water to simulate cool and clammy skin.

Patient: One male (or female) patient. As the patient, you will be required to play the role of a 46-year-old male suffering from abdominal pain. You will be awake and alert and answer all questions. Please read the scenario to familiarize yourself with the information. You will have a fine mist of water sprayed on you to simulate cool and diaphoretic skin.

Instructions

Hi, my name is _____ , and I will be the examiner for this station. This is a hands-on patient assessment station. You will be given information concerning a patient experiencing a medical crisis. You will have all the necessary equipment you need to manage the patient in this station. Please look over the equipment before we go any further. You will be provided with pertinent information only when you ask the appropriate question. For any hands-on procedure, such as auscultation of a blood pressure or breath sounds or taking a pulse, select the appropriate equipment needed (if any) and use the equipment in the manner that it would be used on a patient. I will then give you the relevant clinical data. For example, you must select, place, and begin inflation of the BP cuff before the blood pressure is given to you. I will not answer questions in place of the patient. Therefore, it is imperative that you interact with your patient. Please verbalize to me any signs or symptoms that you find so that I will know you are cognizant of the patient and the patient's clinical appearance.

Scenario

Advise the participant that he is responding to a call of an unknown medical emergency in a middle-class neighborhood at the beginning of his shift. If the participant is a nurse or in-hospital provider, the scenario can be modified to the medical environment—such as reporting to triage after shift change and being told that a patient with abdominal pain has just walked into Medical Room 5. The participant should use the assessment taught in this course.

Initial Impression: 46-year-old male (or female) lying in bed

Scene Size-up/General Impression: Stable patient, no apparent injury noted; there are no scene safety issues present.

Initial Assessment:
> *Mental Status*—A&O × 3, answering questions

> *Airway*—Clear and patent at this time

> *Breathing*—Respirations 28 and labored, crackles in all four lobes

> *Circulation*—Radial pulse at 118 bpm, skin cool and clammy

> *Disability*—Moves all four extremities

Status after Initial Assessment: Stable, potential for deteriorating and becoming a life threat.

Initial Management Priorities: High-flow oxygen at 15 lpm via NRM, cardiac monitor, IV access

Focused History (SAMPLE):
> *Signs and Symptoms*—Pale, cool, clammy skin, lying on his side in distress

> *Allergies*—Penicillin

> *Medications*—Humulin R, Lasix

> *Past Medical History*—IDDM, hypertension

> *Last Oral Intake*—Patient had something last night at dinner, but not much.

> *Events Preceding*—Patient hasn't felt well for a couple of days. When he woke this morning and tried to get out of bed, he almost passed out.

OPQRST:
> *Onset*—Slow

> *Palliation/Provocation*—I felt better when I sat down and didn't move around.

> *Quality*—The pain in my stomach was a dull ache like the flu.

> *Radiation*—It mainly stayed in my stomach.

> *Severity*—Now it's a 5.

> *Time*—It started about 24 hours ago.

Vital Signs:
> *Respirations*—28 and labored, crackles in all four lobes

> *Pulse*—Radial pulse weak at 118 bpm

> *Blood Pressure*—64/42

> *Temperature*—98.4°F (36.9°C)

> *Pulse Oximetry*—Reading error

> *Blood Glucose Level*—72 mg/dl

Focused Physical Exam (Focused Medical Assessment): Unremarkable

Differential/Field Diagnosis: Hypoperfusion (cardiogenic shock)

Management:
1) High-flow oxygen at 15 lpm via NRM

2) IV access × 1, judicious fluid bolus to maintain a systolic pressure between 70–100 mmHg

3) Cardiac monitor—sinus tachycardia with frequent PVCs

4) Dopamine 5–15 µg/kg/min titrated to keep systolic between 70–100 mmHg

5) Rapid transport to appropriate facility

Detailed Physical Exam: En route to appropriate facility if time permits

Ongoing Assessment: There is no change in patient's condition during transport.

Critical Actions:

1) Secure the airway and ensure highest oxygenation at 15 lpm via NRM; if respiratory failure, then PPV.

2) Maintain hemodynamic stability—BP between 70–100 mmHg, no higher.

Teaching Points

1) There are numerous causes and etiologies of hypoperfusion (shock).

2) Always follow an organized approach to rule out possible causes.

3) Diabetic patients often have an altered sensation of pain, so you may not find the classic signs and symptoms of an acute myocardial infarction (AMI).

4) Use of fluid is appropriate because the patient may be volume-depleted because of antihypertensive medications, and the fluid boluses can improve cardiac output based on Starling's Law.

Evaluation

1) *Excellent:* The participant's evaluation of the patient followed set format: initial assessment, focused history (SAMPLE, OPQRST) in an efficient manner. The participant displayed a thorough knowledge of the patient's condition, performed the exam and management in an organized manner, and demonstrated an excellent overall performance.

2) *Good:* The participant's evaluation of the patient followed set format: initial assessment, focused history (SAMPLE, OPQRST) in an acceptable manner with only minor deviation. The participant displayed an above-average knowledge of the patient's condition, performed the exam and management of the patient's condition, and demonstrated an above-average performance.

3) *Fair:* The participant's evaluation of the patient deviated from the set format without causing any further injury to the patient. The participant displayed an average or basic knowledge of the patient's condition and performed an adequate exam and management of the patient's condition.

4) *Inadequate:* The participant's evaluation of the patient deviated significantly from the set format, or the participant's actions endangered the patient's life or significantly exacerbated the condition.

DYSPNEA, RESPIRATORY DISTRESS, OR RESPIRATORY FAILURE

▶ DYSPNEA, RESPIRATORY DISTRESS, OR RESPIRATORY FAILURE: CASE 1

Requirements: One instructor and one patient for every five participants

Prerequisites: Read Chapter 5, "Dyspnea, Respiratory Distress, or Respiratory Failure."

Equipment: One table and chair for the patient to use; jump kit with oxygen supplies (NC, NRM, aerosol mask, PPV device, intubation equipment), stethoscope, BP cuff, cardiac monitor, pulse oximeter, and medication kit with associated medications

Instructor: Your role is vital as your must act as the coordinator of the station and also interact in the scenario. Before the participant arrives at the station, please review the scenario with your patient. For moulage, tint the patient's arms and face with a blue coloring to simulate cyanosis. Then spray the patient's arms with a fine mist of cool water to simulate cool and clammy skin. You will play the spouse of the patient, answering questions for the EMS providers about the condition of your spouse. Please read the scenario to become familiar with the necessary responses. Do not "coach" the participant along during the testing station; rather, allow him to conduct the exam without interruption or help.

Patient: One female (or male) patient. As the patient, you will be required to play the role of a 34-year-old female suffering from difficulty in breathing (DIB). You will be awake and alert, but unable to communicate verbally because of extreme DIB. You should breathe fast (at a rate of 24 per minute) and shallow, exaggerating your respiratory effort by utilizing your diaphragm and neck muscles in an attempt to help you breathe. You will have a fine mist of cold water sprayed onto your arms and face by the instructor to simulate cool and clammy skin. The instructor will act as your spouse and answer all questions that the provider/examiner may have. You can, however, answer yes and no questions by using head gestures. Please read the scenario to familiarize yourself with the information.

Instructions

Hi, my name is _____ , and I will be the examiner for this station. This is a hands-on patient assessment station. You will be given information concerning a patient experiencing a medical crisis. You will have all the necessary equipment you need to manage the patient in this station. Please look over the equipment before we go any further. You will be provided with pertinent information only when you ask the appropriate question. For any hands-on procedure, such as auscultation of a blood pressure or breath sounds or taking a pulse, select the appropriate equipment needed (if any) and use the equipment in the manner that it would be used on a patient. I will then give you the relevant clinical data. For example, you must select, place, and begin inflation of the BP cuff before the blood pressure is given to you. I will not answer questions in place of the patient. Therefore, it is imperative that you interact with

your patient. Please verbalize to me any signs or symptoms that you find so that I will know you are cognizant of the patient and the patient's clinical appearance.

Scenario

Advise the participant that she is responding to an unknown medical emergency. If the participant is a nurse or in-hospital provider, the scenario can be modified to the medical environment—such as the patient sitting in the triage chair with her spouse nearby. The participant should use the assessment taught in this course.

Initial Impression: 34-year-old female (or male) sitting at the kitchen table (or triage desk) hunched forward and leaning on her elbows. The patient is awake, appears pale, and has accessory muscle usage.

Scene Size-up/General Impression: Family escorts you to the patient. The scene is safe for entry and exit. No injury is apparent on brief visual exam. Family members surround patient and are helpful with the history of events.

Initial Assessment:
  Mental Status—Awake, obeys commands

  Airway—Open and patent; no C-spine precautions deemed necessary at this time

  Breathing—Respirations 24 and labored, accessory muscle usage noted in neck, diaphragmatic breathing noted, faint wheezes in upper lobes and absent in bases, patient unable to talk

  Circulation—Very rapid and weak—122 bpm

  Disability—Moves all four extremities.

Status after Initial Assessment: Life threatening; needs immediate intervention

Initial Management Priorities: High-flow oxygen at 15 lpm via NRM, be prepared for possible endotracheal intubation; cardiac monitor, IV access

Focused History (SAMPLE):
  Signs and Symptoms—Respiratory distress, tripod positioning, accessory muscle usage, inability to speak, pulse that fades on inspiration

  NOTE: The participant should ask the spouse questions that require a verbal reply because the patient is unable to communicate except by shaking his head.

  Allergies—Per spouse, penicillin

  Medications—Per spouse, albuterol inhaler that was full this morning now is empty

  Past Medical History—Per spouse, significant only for asthma

  Last Oral Intake—Per spouse, today at lunchtime

  Events Preceding—Per spouse, the patient woke this morning with difficulty breathing. The patient has used her inhaler all day with minimal relief; in fact, the DIB has steadily increased since the morning. When the spouse arrived home, he called EMS because of his wife's condition.

NOTE: The participant should ask the patient to respond with head gestures whenever possible and rely on the spouse for additional information.

OPQRST:

Onset—If the participant utilizes the appropriate questioning, the patient will use head gestures to agree with the description the spouse already gave of the dyspnea steadily increasing all day.

Palliation/Provocation—If the participant utilizes the appropriate questioning, the patient will use head gestures to agree that nothing makes the dyspnea better.

Quality—If the participant utilizes the appropriate questioning, the patient will use head gestures to agree with some type of description such as a "tightness in the chest."

Radiation—If the participant utilizes the appropriate questioning, the patient will use head gestures to answer "no" to any radiation.

Severity—The severity can be inferred from the patient's inability to speak.

Time/Duration—This question has already been answered by the spouse. If the participant utilizes the appropriate questioning, the patient will use head gestures to indicate that she has been treated previously for asthma. If further questioned concerning the severity (Have you ever been intubated because of your asthma?), the patient will shake her head to indicate yes.

Vital Signs:

Respirations—24 and labored

Pulse—Radial 122 bpm that fades on inspiration

Blood Pressure—134/86

Temperature—99.6°F (37.9°C)

Pulse Oximetry—88%

Blood Glucose Level—122 mg/dl

Focused Physical Exam (Focused Medical Assessment): Rapid head-to-toe is unremarkable. Skin tenting is negative. Neurological exam is negative. Lungs are silent in the bases; slight expiratory wheezes in the upper lobes.

Differential/Field Diagnosis: Severe asthma attack

Management:

1) High-flow oxygen at 15 lpm via NRM

2) Nebulized albuterol (or other beta$_2$-specific medication) 2.5 mg treatment

3) Or participant may initiate subcutaneous epinephrine 1:1,000, 0.3–0.5 mg

4) Cardiac monitor—sinus tachycardia with no ectopy

5) IV access at a moderate rate

6) If patient deteriorates, PPV and endotracheal intubation with RSI:

    a) Defasciculating agent—vecuronium 0.01 mg/kg IVP

    b) Sedative—midazolam 0.05–0.1 mg/kg IVP, diazepam 0.2 mg/kg IVP, fentanyl 3–5 mcg/kg, or any of the other sedatives

    c) Cricoid pressure

    d) Succinylcholine 1.5 mg/kg IVP

    e) Intubation

    f) Confirmation

7) Transport

Detailed Physical Exam: En route to appropriate facility as time permits

Ongoing Assessment: Continue to monitor respiratory status. Maintain position of comfort.

Critical Actions:

1) Administer supplemental oxygen before beginning the focused examination. If supplemental oxygen is not applied or not applied in a high concentration (NRM above 12 lpm), then the patient's status should deteriorate into respiratory arrest.

2) If the participant bases his actions on the pulse oximeter reading without any correlation to the patient's signs or symptoms, the patient should deteriorate into respiratory arrest.

Teaching Points

1) Discuss the appearance of patients with DIB—leaning forward and the tripod position help facilitate increased respiratory expansion.

2) Ensure appropriate questioning of the respiratory patient.

3) Discuss the signs of respiratory difficulties—increased respiratory rate and effort, accessory muscle usage, breath sounds and adventitious sounds, increased pulse and BP, pulsus paradoxus, and inability to talk.

4) Don't let past medical history lead you to a diagnosis preemptively.

5) Discuss treatment priorities—early use of high-flow oxygen via NRM, recognition of the possible need for PPV and intubation—because the patient can deteriorate rapidly. Discuss the utilization of RSI to help facilitate endotracheal intubation. Compare and contrast the utilization of beta$_2$-specific bronchial dilators (albuterol, etc.) versus more aggressive treatment with a sympathomimetic such as epinephrine. Discuss steroid use and other drugs such as magnesium sulfate.

6) Explain the advantages and disadvantages of using aerosolized medications on patients with severe bronchial constriction.

Evaluation

1) *Excellent:* The participant's evaluation of the patient followed set format: initial assessment, focused history (SAMPLE, OPQRST) in an efficient manner. The participant displayed a thorough knowledge of the patient's condition, performed the exam and management in an organized manner, and demonstrated an excellent overall performance.

2) *Good:* The participant's evaluation of the patient followed set format: initial assessment, focused history (SAMPLE, OPQRST) in an acceptable manner with only minor deviation. The participant displayed an above-average knowledge of the patient's condition, performed the exam and management of the patient's condition, and demonstrated an above-average performance.

3) *Fair:* The participant's evaluation of the patient deviated from the set format without causing any further injury to the patient. The participant displayed an average or basic knowledge of the patient's condition and performed an adequate exam and management of the patient's condition.

4) *Inadequate:* The participant's evaluation of the patient deviated significantly from the set format, or the participant's actions endangered the patient's life or significantly exacerbated the condition.

▶ DYSPNEA, RESPIRATORY DISTRESS, OR RESPIRATORY FAILURE: CASE 2

Requirements: One instructor and one patient for every five participants

Prerequisites: Read Chapter 5, "Dyspnea, Respiratory Distress, or Respiratory Failure."

Equipment: One table and chair for the patient to use; jump kit with oxygen supplies (NC, NRM, aerosol mask, PPV device, intubation equipment), stethoscope, BP cuff, cardiac monitor, pulse oximeter, and medication kit with associated medications

Instructor: Your role is vital as your must act as the coordinator of the station and also interact in the scenario. Before the participant arrives at the station, please review the scenario with your patient. For moulage, the patient should wear old clothes and have the aroma of alcohol on his breath. The patient should also have a fake blood capsule placed into his mouth to simulate hemoptysis. Please read the scenario to become familiar with the necessary responses. Do not "coach" the participant along during the testing station; rather, allow him to conduct the exam without interruption or help.

Patient: One male (or female) patient. As the patient, you will be required to play the role of a 28-year-old male suffering from difficulty in breathing (DIB). You will be awake and alert and able to communicate. Your respiratory rate will be 32 breaths per minute and shallow. Because you will be simulating a patient with pneumonia, you should cough a couple times every 3 to 4 minutes and break the fake blood capsule when you cough, pretending to have hemoptysis. You live in the city underneath a bridge embankment. City garbage workers heard you coughing and found you beneath a cardboard box that you call "home." Your are in fear of going to the hospital because you think that your "house" may be stolen. You will cooperate with the participant caregiver but with some reluctance. Please read the scenario to familiarize yourself with all the information.

Instructions

Hi, my name is _____ , and I will be the examiner for this station. This is a hands-on patient assessment station. You will be given information concerning a patient experiencing a medical crisis. You will have all the necessary equipment you need to manage the patient in this station. Please look over the equipment before we go any further. You will be provided with pertinent information only when you ask the appropriate question. For any hands-on procedure, such as auscultation of a blood pressure or breath sounds or taking a pulse, select the appropriate equipment needed (if any) and use the equipment in the manner that it would be used on a patient. I will then give you the relevant clinical data. For example, you must select, place, and begin inflation of the BP cuff before the blood pressure is given to you. I will not answer questions in place of the patient. Therefore, it is imperative that you interact with your patient. Please verbalize to me any signs or symptoms that you find so that I will know you are cognizant of the patient and the patient's clinical appearance.

Scenario

Advise the participant that he is responding to a call for difficulty in breathing in the "old section of town." If the participant is a nurse or in-hospital provider, the scenario can be modified to the medical environment—such as the police department brings a homeless man to triage for evaluation. The participant should use the assessment taught in this course.

Initial Impression: 28-year-old male (or female) coughing excessively, A&O × 3, resistant to authority

Scene Size-up/General Impression: The police escort you to the patient. The scene is safe for entry and exit. No injury is apparent on brief visual exam. Garbage workers describe what they found.

Initial Assessment:

Mental Status—Awake, obeys commands reluctantly

Airway—Open and patent, no C-spine precautions deemed necessary at this time, productive cough, blood-stained sputum

Breathing—Respirations 32 and labored, breath sounds diminished in right lower lobe with wheezes in upper right and left lobes

Circulation—Radial pulse strong at 98 bpm, skin warm and dry to touch

Disability—Moves all four extremities

Status after Initial Assessment: Not immediately life threatening, stable but potentially serious

Initial Management Priorities: Oxygen at 2–4 lpm via nasal cannula, cardiac monitor, IV access

Focused History (SAMPLE):

Signs and Symptoms—Respiratory distress, a cough producing small amounts of blood, and a possible fever

Allergies—Some pain shot

Medications—None besides occasional illicit drug use

Past Medical History—None that the patient reports

Last Oral Intake—A couple of days ago at the soup kitchen

Events Preceding—Patient states he caught a cold when the temperature dipped below 32°F (0°C) and was never able to shake it. The cold went to his chest, and he began to cough up green and reddish sputum.

OPQRST:

Onset—It started about two weeks ago, getting worse 3 to 4 days ago.

Palliation/Provocation—When I cough it hurts real bad in my chest.

Quality—There's a sharp pain when I take a deep breath.

Radiation—None

Severity—I don't have any energy anymore; I feel worn out all the time.

Time/Duration—I already told you that for the past 3 to 4 days it's been getting worse.

Vital Signs:

    Respirations—32 and labored and shallow

    Pulse—Radial pulse regular at 98 bpm

    Blood Pressure—114/62

    Temperature—101.4°F (38.9°C)

    Pulse Oximetry—93%

    Blood Glucose Level—92 mg/dl

Focused Physical Exam (Focused Medical Assessment): Possible needle track on arms. Patient appears to have poor hygiene.

Differential/Field Diagnosis: Pneumonia—mainly localized to right lower lobe

Management:

1) Emotional reassurance to gain patient's confidence

2) Oxygen by nasal cannula at 2–4 lpm if patient will tolerate

3) Cardiac monitor

4) IV access—possible rehydration if protocol allows

5) Nebulized albuterol (or other beta$_2$-specific medication) 2.5 mg treatment

Detailed Physical Exam: En route to appropriate facility if time permits

Ongoing Assessment: There is no change in patient's condition during transport.

Critical Actions: Gain patient's confidence and convince him to come to the ED for evaluation.

Teaching Points

1) Discuss the appearance of patients with DIB—mild versus severe.

2) Ensure appropriate questioning of the respiratory patient.

3) Discuss the signs of respiratory difficulties—increased respiratory rate and coughing with productive sputum.

4) Don't let past medical history lead you to a diagnosis preemptively.

5) Discuss treatment priorities—early use of low-flow oxygen and aerosolized medications for pneumonia patients.

Evaluation

1) *Excellent:* The participant's evaluation of the patient followed set format: initial assessment, focused history (SAMPLE, OPQRST) in an efficient manner. The participant displayed a thorough knowledge of the patient's condition, performed the exam and management in an organized manner, and demonstrated an excellent overall performance.

2) *Good:* The participant's evaluation of the patient followed set format: initial assessment, focused history (SAMPLE, OPQRST) in an acceptable manner with only minor deviation. The participant displayed an above-average knowledge of the patient's condition, performed the exam and management of the patient's condition, and demonstrated an above-average performance.

3) *Fair:* The participant's evaluation of the patient deviated from the set format without causing any further injury to the patient. The participant displayed an average or basic knowledge of the patient's condition and performed an adequate exam and management of the patient's condition.

4) *Inadequate:* The participant's evaluation of the patient deviated significantly from the set format, or the participant's actions endangered the patient's life or significantly exacerbated the condition.

▶ DYSPNEA, RESPIRATORY DISTRESS, OR RESPIRATORY FAILURE: CASE 3

Requirements: One instructor and one patient for every five participants

Prerequisites: Read Chapter 5, "Dyspnea, Respiratory Distress, or Respiratory Failure."

Equipment: One table and chair for the patient to use; jump kit with oxygen supplies (NC, NRM, aerosol mask, PPV device, intubation equipment), stethoscope, BP cuff, cardiac monitor, pulse oximeter, and medication kit with associated medications

Instructor: Your role is vital as your must act as the coordinator of the station and also interact in the scenario. Before the participant arrives at the station, please review the scenario with your patient. For moulage, tint the patient's arms and face with a blue coloring to simulate cyanosis. Then spray the patient's arms with a fine mist of cool water to simulate cool and clammy skin. You will play the son or daughter of the patient and answer questions for the participant concerning why you called EMS. You will reply that you awoke early this morning because the house was "ice cold." You went to your mother's room to close the window, noticed her condition, and called EMS. Please read the scenario to become familiar with the necessary responses. Do not "coach" the participant along during the testing station; rather, allow him to conduct the exam without interruption or help.

Patient: One female (or male) patient. As the patient, you will be required to play the role of a 78-year-old female suffering from difficulty in breathing (DIB). You will be awake and alert and able to communicate in short sentences. You should breathe fast (at a rate of 32 per minute) and shallow, exaggerating your respiratory effort by using your diaphragm and neck muscles in an attempt to help you breathe. You will have a fine mist of cold water sprayed onto your arms and face by the instructor to simulate cool, clammy skin. The instructor will act as you son or daughter. If questioned about the history behind the mild DIB, you will answer that you had mild DIB before bedtime. You woke very anxious and moderately short of breath, having to prop two pillows under your back and open the window just to breathe. You have had two past myocardial infarctions. You currently take digoxin (Lanoxin), furosemide (Lasix), prazosin (Minipress), and potassium supplements (Kaochlor). If questioned about when you last took your medications, hesitantly reply that you ran out of your water pill two weeks ago and haven't had the money to refill it since. Remember that you are short of breath, so you need to answer questions in short, broken sentences, pausing often to catch your breath. Please read the scenario to familiarize yourself with the information.

Instructions

Hi, my name is _____ , and I will be the examiner for this station. This is a hands-on patient assessment station. You will be given information concerning a patient experiencing a medical crisis. You will have all the necessary equipment you need to manage the patient in this station. Please look over the equipment before we go any further. You will be provided with pertinent information only when you ask the appropriate question. For any hands-on procedure, such as auscultation of a blood pressure or breath sounds or taking a pulse, select the appropriate equipment needed (if any) and use the equipment in the manner that it would be used on a patient. I will then give you the relevant clinical data. For example, you must select, place, and begin inflation of the BP cuff before the blood pressure is given to you. I will not answer questions in place of the patient. Therefore, it is imperative that you interact with your patient. Please verbalize to me any signs or symptoms that you find so that I will know you are cognizant of the patient and the patient's clinical appearance.

Scenario

Advise the participant that she is responding to a call of shortness of breath. If the participant is a nurse or in-hospital provider, the scenario can be modified to the medical environment—such as the triage nurse brings a patient who is short of breath to Medical Room 1. The participant should use the assessment taught in this course.

Initial Impression: 78-year-old female (or male) sitting in bed at home or in ED, leaning forward with two to three pillows propped up behind her. The patient is awake, very anxious, appears pale, and has accessory muscle usage.

Scene Size-up/General Impression: The scene is safe for entry and exit. No injury is apparent on brief visual exam. Son describes what he found.

Initial Assessment:
  Mental Status—Awake, obeys commands, anxious

  Airway—Patent, with some foamy saliva present

  Breathing—Respirations 32 and labored, accessory muscle usage noted in neck, diaphragmatic breathing noted, lung sounds in the bases are predominately rales and rhonchi with wheezes bilaterally in the upper lobes, patient unable to talk in complete sentences

  Circulation—Radial pulse irregular at 105 bpm, skin cool and clammy

  Disability—Moves all four extremities

Status after Initial Assessment: Potentially life threatening.

Initial Management Priorities: High-flow oxygen at 15 lpm via NRM, cardiac monitor, IV access, position of comfort

Focused History (SAMPLE):
  Signs and Symptoms—Respiratory distress, leaning forward with pillows behind her, accessory muscle usage, inability to speak in complete sentences

  Allergies—NKA

  Medications—Lanoxin, Lasix, Minipress, Kaochlor

  Past Medical History—Two previous MIs and atrial fibrillation

  Last Oral Intake—A bowl of potato chips before bedtime

  Events Preceding—Began to have mild DIB before going to bed. The patient awoke by an inability to breathe that was almost suffocating. The patient opened the window to let in some cool air and propped herself up with two pillows. When her son awoke because of the cold chill, he found her in severe respiratory distress and called EMS.

OPQRST:

Onset—I've been mildly short of breath for the past few days, and it got worse this evening.

Palliation/Provocation—When I sit forward, it feels as if I can catch my breath. If I lie flat, I feel like I'm suffocating.

Quality—It feels like I'm suffocating, like heaviness in my lungs.

Radiation—None, just the heaviness in my lungs.

Severity—I can't sleep, can't lie down, can't even talk without becoming winded.

Time/Duration—I told you that it's been getting worse for a few days. (If the participant asks about past episodes of respiratory failure and whether or not the patient has ever had to be intubated before, the reply will be yes.)

Vital Signs:

Respirations—32 and labored and shallow

Pulse—Radial pulse irregular at 105 bpm *(If monitor is placed on patient, it will show atrial fibrillation.)*

Blood Pressure—168/102

Temperature—99.8°F (38.0°C)

Pulse Oximetry—91%

Blood Glucose Level—128 mg/dl

Focused Physical Exam (Focused Medical Assessment): Bilateral 3+ pitting edema to the ankles

Differential/Field Diagnosis: Congestive heart failure with acute pulmonary edema

Management:

1) High-flow oxygen at 15 lpm via NRM

2) Nitroglycerin sublingual 0.4 mg

3) Cardiac monitor—atrial fibrillation

4) IV access

5) Lasix 0.5—1.0 mg/kg IVP

6) Morphine sulfate 2–4 mg IVP—watch for respiratory depression

7) Nebulized albuterol (or other beta$_2$-specific medication) 2.5 mg treatment

8) If patient deteriorates, then PPV and endotracheal intubation with RSI:

   a) Defasciculating agent—vecuronium 0.01 mg/kg IVP

   b) Sedative—midazolam 0.05–0.1 mg/kg IVP, diazepam 0.2 mg/kg IVP, fentanyl 3–5 mcg/kg, or any of the other sedatives

   c) Cricoid pressure

    d) Succinylcholine 1.5 mg/kg IVP

    e) Intubation

    f) Confirmation

Detailed Physical Exam: En route to appropriate facility as time permits

Ongoing Assessment: Continue to monitor respiratory status. Maintain position of comfort.

Critical Actions:

1) Administer supplemental oxygen before beginning the focused examination. If supplemental oxygen is not applied or not applied in a high concentration (NRM above 12 lpm), then the patient's status should deteriorate into respiratory arrest.

2) If the participant bases his actions on the pulse oximeter reading without any correlation to the patient's signs or symptoms, the patient should deteriorate into respiratory arrest.

Teaching Points

1) Discuss the appearance of patients with DIB—leaning forward, using multiple pillows to sleep.

2) Ensure appropriate questioning of the respiratory patient.

3) Discuss the signs of respiratory difficulties—increased respiratory rate and effort, accessory muscle usage, breath sounds and adventitious sounds, increased pulse and BP, and inability to talk in complete sentences.

4) Don't let past medical history lead you to a diagnosis preemptively.

5) Discuss treatment priorities—early use of high-flow oxygen via NRM, recognition of the possible need for PPV and intubation—because the patient can deteriorate rapidly. Discuss the utilization of RSI to help facilitate endotracheal intubation.

6) Review the indications of nitroglycerin, morphine, and Lasix in the management of this patient.

Evaluation

1) *Excellent:* The participant's evaluation of the patient followed set format: initial assessment, focused history (SAMPLE, OPQRST) in an efficient manner. The participant displayed a thorough knowledge of the patient's condition, performed the exam and management in an organized manner, and demonstrated an excellent overall performance.

2) *Good:* The participant's evaluation of the patient followed set format: initial assessment, focused history (SAMPLE, OPQRST) in an acceptable manner with only minor deviation. The participant displayed an above-average knowledge of the patient's condition, performed the exam and management of the patient's condition, and demonstrated an above-average performance.

3) *Fair:* The participant's evaluation of the patient deviated from the set format without causing any further injury to the patient. The participant displayed an average or basic knowledge of the patient's condition and performed an adequate exam and management of the patient's condition.

4) *Inadequate:* The participant's evaluation of the patient deviated significantly from the set format, or the participant's actions endangered the patient's life or significantly exacerbated the condition.

▶ Dyspnea, Respiratory Distress, or Respiratory Failure: Case 4

Requirements: One instructor and one patient for every five participants

Prerequisites: Read Chapter 5, "Dyspnea, Respiratory Distress, or Respiratory Failure."

Equipment: One table and chair for the patient to use; jump kit with oxygen supplies (NC, NRM, aerosol mask, PPV device, intubation equipment), stethoscope, BP cuff, cardiac monitor, pulse oximeter, and medication kit with associated medications

Instructor: Your role is vital as your must act as the coordinator of the station and also interact in the scenario. Before the participant arrives at the station, please review the scenario with your patient. For moulage, tint the patient's arms and face with a blue coloring to simulate cyanosis. Then spray the patient's arms with a fine mist of cool water to simulate cool and clammy skin. Please read the scenario to become familiar with the necessary responses. Do not "coach" the participant along during the testing station; rather, allow him to conduct the exam without interruption or help.

Patient: One male (or female) patient. As the patient, you will be required to play the role of a 28-year-old male suffering from difficulty in breathing (DIB). You will be awake and alert and able to communicate in short sentences. You should breathe fast (at a rate of 28 per minute) and shallow, exaggerating your respiratory effort by using your diaphragm and neck muscles in an attempt to help you breathe. To make the scenario as realistic as possible, cough frequently, attempting to clear out your airway. You will have a fine mist of cold water sprayed onto your arms and face by the instructor to simulate diaphoresis. Remember that you are short of breath, so you need to answer questions in short, broken sentences, pausing often to catch your breath. You have a past history of asthma, which requires you to use an inhaler three times a day. Please read the scenario to familiarize yourself with the information.

Instructions

Hi, my name is _____ , and I will be the examiner for this station. This is a hands-on patient assessment station. You will be given information concerning a patient experiencing a medical crisis. You will have all the necessary equipment you need to manage the patient in this station. Please look over the equipment before we go any further. You will be provided with pertinent information only when you ask the appropriate question. For any hands-on procedure, such as auscultation of a blood pressure or breath sounds or taking a pulse, select the appropriate equipment needed (if any) and use the equipment in the manner that it would be used on a patient. I will then give you the relevant clinical data. For example, you must select, place, and begin inflation of the BP cuff before the blood pressure is given to you. I will not answer questions in place of the patient. Therefore, it is imperative that you interact with your patient. Please verbalize to me any signs or symptoms that you find so that I will know you are cognizant of the patient and the patient's clinical appearance.

Scenario

Advise the participant that he is responding to a call of difficulty in breathing at the county fair. If the participant is a nurse or in-hospital provider, the scenario can be modified to the medical environment—such as the triage nurse brings a patient who has difficulty breathing to Medical Room 1. The participant should use the assessment taught in this course.

Initial Impression: 28-year-old male (or female) sitting up and in obvious respiratory distress. The patient is awake, very anxious, appears cyanotic, and has accessory muscle usage.

Scene Size-up/General Impression: The scene is safe for entry and exit. No injury is apparent on brief visual exam.

Initial Assessment:

Mental Status—Awake, obeys commands, anxious

Airway—Patent

Breathing—Respirations 28 and shallow, accessory muscle usage noted in neck, diaphragmatic breathing noted, lung sounds in the bases absent with wheezes in the apexes

Circulation—Radial pulse regular and bounding at 103 bpm, skin warm and clammy

Disability—Moves all four extremities

Status after Initial Assessment: Serious, potentially life threatening.

Initial Management Priorities: High-flow oxygen at 15 lpm via NRM, cardiac monitor, IV access, position of comfort

Focused History (SAMPLE):

Signs and Symptoms—Respiratory distress, leaning forward in a tripod position, peripheral cyanosis, accessory muscle usage, inability to speak in complete sentences

Allergies—Grass, pollen, and dust

Medications—Atrovent inhaler

Past Medical History—Hospitalization for "bad asthma attack." (If specifically asked, intubated for asthma attack in past.)

Last Oral Intake—Lunchtime

Events Preceding—Patient has been at the fair all day, feeding the horses and cleaning the stalls.

OPQRST:

Onset—It started right after lunch, about 2 hours ago.

Palliation/Provocation—If I lie down, I know I'll stop breathing.

Quality—It feels like I can't get any air in.

Radiation—None

Severity—One of the worst attacks ever.

Time/Duration—It started about 2 hours ago, and I haven't been able to stop it with my inhaler. In fact, it's been getting worse.

Vital Signs:

Respirations—28 and labored and shallow

Pulse—Radial pulse irregular at 103 bpm and bounding

Blood Pressure—104/72

Temperature—99.8°F (38.0°C)

Pulse Oximetry—88%

Blood Glucose Level—118 mg/dl

Focused Physical Exam (Focused Medical Assessment): Peripheral cyanosis that is getting worse

Differential/Field Diagnosis: Acute exacerbation of asthma

Management:

1) High-flow oxygen at 15 lpm via NRM

2) Cardiac monitor—sinus tachycardia with unifocal PVCs (4 per minute)

3) Nebulized albuterol (or other beta$_2$-specific medication) 2.5 mg treatment

4) IV access

5) Consider use of epinephrine IV if patient's condition does not improve, dosage 0.3–0.5 mg 1:10,000 IVP.

6) Consider fluid challenge to increase pressure.

7) If patient deteriorates, PPV and endotracheal intubation with RSI:

   a) Defasciculating agent—vecuronium 0.01 mg/kg IVP

   b) Sedative—midazolam 0.05–0.1 mg/kg IVP, diazepam 0.2 mg/kg IVP, fentanyl 3–5 mcg/kg, or any of the other sedatives

   c) Cricoid pressure

   d) Succinylcholine 1.5 mg/kg IVP

   e) Intubation

   f) Confirmation

Detailed Physical Exam: En route to appropriate facility as time permits

Ongoing Assessment: Continue to monitor for respiratory distress. Maintain position of comfort.

Critical Actions:

1) Administer supplemental oxygen before beginning the focused examination. If supplemental oxygen is not applied or not applied in a high concentration (NRM above 12 lpm), then the patient's status should deteriorate into respiratory arrest.

2) If the participant bases his actions on the pulse oximeter reading without any correlation to the patient's signs or symptoms, the patient should deteriorate into respiratory arrest.

Teaching Points

1) Discuss the appearance of patients with DIB—leaning forward tripod position.

2) Discuss the appearance of peripheral versus central cyanosis.

3) Ensure appropriate questioning of the respiratory patient.

4) Discuss the signs of respiratory difficulties—increased respiratory rate and effort, accessory muscle usage, breath sounds and adventitious sounds, increased pulse and BP, and inability to talk in complete sentences.

5) Don't let past medical history lead you to a diagnosis preemptively.

6) Discuss treatment priorities—early use of high-flow oxygen via NRM, recognition of the possible need for PPV and intubation—because the patient can deteriorate rapidly. Discuss the utilization of RSI to help facilitate endotracheal intubation.

7) Review the indications for fluid resuscitation and other medications such as steroids and magnesium sulfate or other asthma management pharmacological tools.

Evaluation

1) *Excellent:* The participant's evaluation of the patient followed set format: initial assessment, focused history (SAMPLE, OPQRST) in an efficient manner. The participant displayed a thorough knowledge of the patient's condition, performed the exam and management in an organized manner, and demonstrated an excellent overall performance.

2) *Good:* The participant's evaluation of the patient followed set format: initial assessment, focused history (SAMPLE, OPQRST) in an acceptable manner with only minor deviation. The participant displayed an above-average knowledge of the patient's condition, performed the exam and management of the patient's condition, and demonstrated an above-average performance.

3) *Fair:* The participant's evaluation of the patient deviated from the set format without causing any further injury to the patient. The participant displayed an average or basic knowledge of the patient's condition and performed an adequate exam and management of the patient's condition.

4) *Inadequate:* The participant's evaluation of the patient deviated significantly from the set format, or the participant's actions endangered the patient's life or significantly exacerbated the condition.

⊞ CHEST PAIN

▶ CHEST PAIN: CASE 1

Requirements: One instructor and one patient for every five participants

Prerequisites: Read Chapter 6, "Chest Pain."

Equipment: One table and chair for the patient to use; jump kit with oxygen supplies (NC, NRM, aerosol mask, PPV device, intubation equipment), stethoscope, BP cuff, cardiac monitor, pulse oximeter, and medication kit with associated medications

Instructor: Your role is vital as your must act as the coordinator of the station and also interact in the scenario. Before the participant arrives at the station, please review the scenario with your patient. For moulage, tint the patient's arms and face to simulate being pale. Please read the scenario to become familiar with the necessary responses. Do not "coach" the participant along during the testing station; rather, allow him to conduct the exam without interruption or help.

Patient: One female (or male) patient. As the patient, you will be required to play the role of a 33-year-old female suffering from chest pain. You were moving a couch when you felt a sharp pain in your left chest and experienced difficulty breathing. Please read the scenario to familiarize yourself with the information.

Instructions

Hi, my name is _____ , and I will be the examiner for this station. This is a hands-on patient assessment station. You will be given information concerning a patient experiencing a medical crisis. You will have all the necessary equipment you need to manage the patient in this station. Please look over the equipment before we go any further. You will be provided with pertinent information only when you ask the appropriate question. For any hands-on procedure, such as auscultation of a blood pressure or breath sounds or taking a pulse, select the appropriate equipment needed (if any) and use the equipment in the manner that it would be used on a patient. I will then give you the relevant clinical data. For example, you must select, place, and begin inflation of the BP cuff before the blood pressure is given to you. I will not answer questions in place of the patient. Therefore, it is imperative that you interact with your patient. Please verbalize to me any signs or symptoms that you find so that I will know you are cognizant of the patient and the patient's clinical appearance.

Scenario

Advise the participant that she is responding to a call of chest pain. If the participant is a nurse or in-hospital provider, the scenario can be modified to the medical environment—such as the patient walked into triage complaining of chest pain. The participant should use the assessment taught in this course.

Initial Impression: 33-year-old female (or male) sitting on the porch/triage desk leaning forward and visibly agitated.

Scene Size-up/General Impression: The scene is safe for entry and exit. No injury is apparent on brief visual exam. At the scene, you see a moving van parked in the front yard.

Initial Assessment:

Mental Status—Responsive and visibly agitated, A&O × 3

Airway—Open and clear

Breathing—Respirations 22 and regular, breath sounds diminished on the left

Circulation—Radial pulse regular 102 bpm; skin warm, dry, and pale

Disability—Moves all four extremities

Status after Initial Assessment: Serious, potentially life threatening. May need immediate intervention.

Initial Management Priorities: High-flow oxygen at 15 lpm via NRM, cardiac monitor, IV access, position of comfort

Focused History (SAMPLE):

Signs and Symptoms—Agitated, chest pain, DIB, diminished breath sounds on left

Allergies—NKA

Medications—Patient denies any

Past Medical History—Patient denies

Last Oral Intake—About an hour ago, hot dog and chips

Events Preceding—The patient explains that she was moving the couch when she felt a sudden sharp pain in her left chest and experienced difficulty breathing.

OPQRST:

Onset—It was very rapid.

Palliation/Provocation—I can't catch my breath if I lie down.

Quality—At first it was sharp; now it's a dull, constant ache.

Radiation—Throughout my chest

Severity—On a scale of 1 to 10, it's a 7.

Time/Duration—It started approximately 30 minutes ago.

Vital Signs:

Respirations—22 and regular

Pulse—Radial pulse at 102 bpm

Blood Pressure—146/92

Temperature—99.2°F (37.6°C)

Pulse Oximetry—92%

Blood Glucose Level—112 mg/dl

Focused Physical Exam (Focused Medical Assessment): Rapid head-to-toe is unremarkable. Patient is visibly agitated.

Differential/Field Diagnosis: Spontaneous simple pneumothorax

Management:

1) High-flow oxygen at 15 lpm via NRM

2) IV access

3) Cardiac monitor—sinus tachycardia with no ectopy

4) Transport to the appropriate facility

5) Continued monitoring for the potential of a tension pneumothorax

Detailed Physical Exam: En route to appropriate facility if time permits

Ongoing Assessment: There is no change in patient's condition during transport.

Critical Actions:

1) Secure airway and ensure highest oxygenation at 15 lpm via NRM.

2) Allow the patient to assume position of comfort for breathing; do not force the patient to lie supine.

Teaching Points

1) There are numerous causes and etiologies of chest pain. Assist the participant in classifying chest pain to body system and causes (e.g., cardiac vs. respiratory, trauma vs. medical) for rule outs.

2) Always follow an organized approach to rule out possible causes.

3) Compare and contrast clinical findings of a simple pneumothorax and a tension pneumothorax.

4) Compare and contrast the treatment of a simple and a tension pneumothorax.

Evaluation

1) *Excellent:* The participant's evaluation of the patient followed set format: initial assessment, focused history (SAMPLE, OPQRST) in an efficient manner. The participant displayed a thorough knowledge of the patient's condition, performed the exam and management in an organized manner, and demonstrated an excellent overall performance.

2) *Good:* The participant's evaluation of the patient followed set format: initial assessment, focused history (SAMPLE, OPQRST) in an acceptable manner with only minor deviation. The participant displayed an above-average knowledge of the patient's condition, performed the exam and management of the patient's condition, and demonstrated an above-average performance.

3) *Fair:* The participant's evaluation of the patient deviated from the set format without causing any further injury to the patient. The participant displayed an average or basic knowledge of the patient's condition and performed an adequate exam and management of the patient's condition.

4) *Inadequate:* The participant's evaluation of the patient deviated significantly from the set format, or the participant's actions endangered the patient's life or significantly exacerbated the condition.

▶ CHEST PAIN: CASE 2

Requirements: One instructor and one patient for every five participants

Prerequisites: Read Chapter 6, "Chest Pain."

Equipment: One table and chair for the patient to use; jump kit with oxygen supplies (NC, NRM, aerosol mask, PPV device, intubation equipment), stethoscope, BP cuff, cardiac monitor, pulse oximeter, and medication kit with associated medications

Instructor: Your role is vital as your must act as the coordinator of the station and also interact in the scenario. Before the participant arrives at the station, please review the scenario with your patient. You also will act as the nurse who is responsible for this patient. Please read the scenario to become familiar with the necessary responses. Do not "coach" the participant along during the testing station; rather, allow him to conduct the exam without interruption or help.

Patient: One male (or female) patient. As the patient, you will be required to play the role of a 74-year-old male suffering from chest pain. You will be awake and alert and able to answer all questions. The pain is a burning pain in your back and jaw that started about three days earlier and has not gotten any better. Please read the scenario to familiarize yourself with all the information.

Instructions

Hi, my name is _____ , and I will be the examiner for this station. This is a hands-on patient assessment station. You will be given information concerning a patient experiencing a medical crisis. You will have all the necessary equipment you need to manage the patient in this station. Please look over the equipment before we go any further. You will be provided with pertinent information only when you ask the appropriate question. For any hands-on procedure, such as auscultation of a blood pressure or breath sounds or taking a pulse, select the appropriate equipment needed (if any) and use the equipment in the manner that it would be used on a patient. I will then give you the relevant clinical data. For example, you must select, place, and begin inflation of the BP cuff before the blood pressure is given to you. I will not answer questions in place of the patient. Therefore, it is imperative that you interact with your patient. Please verbalize to me any signs or symptoms that you find so that I will know you are cognizant of the patient and the patient's clinical appearance.

Scenario

Advise the participant that he is responding to a nursing home for a chest pain call. If the participant is a nurse or in-hospital provider, the scenario can be modified to the medical environment—such as the patient has walked into the ED and collapsed in the triage seat. The participant should use the assessment taught in this course.

Initial Impression: 74-year-old male (or female) nursing home patient sitting in a chair.

Scene Size-up/General Impression: The scene is safe for entry and exit. No injury is apparent on brief visual exam. Nursing staff directs you to the patient.

Initial Assessment:

Mental Status—Awake, alert, answering all questions

Airway—Clear and patent

Breathing—Respirations 32 and very shallow

Circulation—Radial pulse 104 bpm and irregular, skin very warm and dry to touch

Disability—Moves all four extremities

Status after Initial Assessment: Not immediately life threatening; stable but potentially serious

Initial Management Priorities: High-flow oxygen at 15 lpm via NRM, cardiac monitor, IV access

Focused History (SAMPLE):

Signs and Symptoms—Chest pain, difficulty breathing, skin warm to touch

Allergies—Sulfa drugs

Medications—One aspirin a day, digoxin, Coumadin

Past Medical History—Atrial fibrillation

Last Oral Intake—At lunchtime

Events Preceding—Patient's chest has been hurting for the past 3 to 4 days, and he couldn't get in to see his doctor.

OPQRST:

Onset—It started slowly about 3 to 4 days ago.

Palliation/Provocation—I can't sleep at night because my chest really hurts if I lie down.

Quality—It's a burning pain that just won't go away.

Radiation—It kind of goes into may back and jaw.

Severity—On a scale of 1 to 10, it's a 6.

Time/Duration—It's been 3 to 4 days.

Vital Signs:

Respirations—32 and shallow

Pulse—Radial pulse rapid and irregular at 104 bpm

Blood Pressure—142/67

Temperature—102.6°F (39.5°C)

Pulse Oximetry—93%

Blood Glucose Level—138 mg/dl

Focused Physical Exam (Focused Medical Assessment): (*If participant asks, the patient has a "rubbing" heart sound.*) Atrial fibrillation on the monitor. (*If the participant asks, ST-segment depression throughout leads, without localization.*)

Differential/Field Diagnosis: Pericarditis

Management:

1) Supplemental oxygen at 15 lpm via NRM

2) IV access

3) Cardiac monitor—artrial fibrillation (*If participant asks, there is ST-segment depression throughout leads, without localization.*)

4) Transport

Detailed Physical Exam: En route to appropriate facility if time permits

Ongoing Assessment: There is no change in patient's condition during transport.

Critical Actions:

1) Secure airway and ensure highest oxygenation at 15 lpm via NRM.

2) Do not force patient to lie on the cot.

Teaching Points

1) There are numerous causes and etiologies of chest pain. Assist the participant in classifying chest pain to body system and causes (e.g., cardiac vs. respiratory, trauma vs. medical) for rule outs.

2) Always follow an organized approach to rule out possible causes.

3) Compare and contrast clinical findings of an AMI to pericarditis. Not all chest pain is an AMI.

4) Pericarditis usually will not respond to morphine sulfate or nitro administration. When in doubt, treat as an AMI.

Evaluation

1) *Excellent:* The participant's evaluation of the patient followed set format: initial assessment, focused history (SAMPLE, OPQRST) in an efficient manner. The participant displayed a thorough knowledge of the patient's condition, performed the exam and management in an organized manner, and demonstrated an excellent overall performance.

2) *Good:* The participant's evaluation of the patient followed set format: initial assessment, focused history (SAMPLE, OPQRST) in an acceptable manner with only minor deviation. The participant displayed an above-average knowledge of the patient's condition, performed the exam and management of the patient's condition, and demonstrated an above-average performance.

3) *Fair:* The participant's evaluation of the patient deviated from the set format without causing any further injury to the patient. The participant displayed an average or basic knowledge of the patient's condition and performed an adequate exam and management of the patient's condition.

4) *Inadequate:* The participant's evaluation of the patient deviated significantly from the set format, or the participant's actions endangered the patient's life or significantly exacerbated the condition.

▶ CHEST PAIN: CASE 3

Requirements: One instructor and one patient for every five participants

Prerequisites: Read Chapter 6, "Chest Pain."

Equipment: One table and chair for the patient to use; jump kit with oxygen supplies (NC, NRM, aerosol mask, PPV device, intubation equipment), stethoscope, BP cuff, cardiac monitor, pulse oximeter, and medication kit with associated medications

Instructor: Your role is vital as your must act as the coordinator of the station and also interact in the scenario. Before the participant arrives at the station, please review the scenario with your patient. Spray the patient's arms with a fine mist of cool water to simulate cool and clammy skin. Please read the scenario to become familiar with the necessary responses. Do not "coach" the participant along during the testing station; rather, allow him to conduct the exam without interruption or help.

Patient: One female (or male) patient. As the patient, you will be required to play the role of a 46-year-old female suffering from chest pain. You will be awake and alert and clutching your chest because of the intense pain. Please read the scenario to familiarize yourself with the information.

Instructions

Hi, my name is _____ , and I will be the examiner for this station. This is a hands-on patient assessment station. You will be given information concerning a patient experiencing a medical crisis. You will have all the necessary equipment you need to manage the patient in this station. Please look over the equipment before we go any further. You will be provided with pertinent information only when you ask the appropriate question. For any hands-on procedure, such as auscultation of a blood pressure or breath sounds or taking a pulse, select the appropriate equipment needed (if any) and use the equipment in the manner that it would be used on a patient. I will then give you the relevant clinical data. For example, you must select, place, and begin inflation of the BP cuff before the blood pressure is given to you. I will not answer questions in place of the patient. Therefore, it is imperative that you interact with your patient. Please verbalize to me any signs or symptoms that you find so that I will know you are cognizant of the patient and the patient's clinical appearance.

Scenario

Advise the participant that she is responding to an unknown medical emergency in a middle-class neighborhood. If the participant is a nurse or in-hospital provider, the scenario can be modified to the medical environment—such as the triage nurse brings a patient who complains of "not feeling well" to Medical Room 1. The participant should use the assessment taught in this course.

Initial Impression: 46-year-old female (or male) lying on the couch, clutching her (his) chest

Scene Size-up/General Impression: The scene is safe for entry and exit. No injury is apparent on brief visual exam.

Initial Assessment:

Mental Status—A&O × 3, answering questions

Airway—Clear and patent at this time

Breathing—Respirations 28

Circulation—Radial pulse irregular at 62 bpm, skin cool and clammy

Disability—Moves all four extremities

Status after Initial Assessment: Critical, potentially life threatening

Initial Management Priorities: High-flow oxygen at 15 lpm via NRM, cardiac monitor, IV access

Focused History (SAMPLE):

Signs and Symptoms—Pale, cool, clammy skin; clutching her chest

Allergies—NKA

Medications—Isosorbide, Lasix

Past Medical History—Past MI and hypertension

Last Oral Intake—Patient states she had something last night at dinner, but not much.

Events Preceding—When patient woke this morning, she tried to get off the couch and almost passed out from the chest pain. The pain didn't go away, so she called 911.

OPQRST:

Onset—It was there when I woke this morning.

Palliation/Provocation—The pain is not as bad if I don't move around.

Quality—A pressure in my chest

Radiation—It does go into my neck.

Severity—On a scale of 1 to 10, it's an 8.

Time/Duration—Since I called you

Vital Signs:

Respirations—28

Pulse—Radial pulse irregular at 62 bpm *(If monitor is placed on patient, it will show sinus bradycardia with frequent PVCs and ST elevation.)*

Blood Pressure—106/42

Temperature—98.4°F (37°C)

Pulse Oximetry—95%

Blood Glucose Level—106 mg/dl

Focused Physical Exam (Focused Medical Assessment): Nothing significant

Differential/Field Diagnosis: Acute myocardial infarction (AMI)

Management:
1) High-flow oxygen at 15 lpm via NRM

2) IV access

3) Cardiac monitor—sinus bradycardia with frequent PVCs and ST elevation. *(If the participant asks, the pain is the same as when patient had his last MI.)*

4) Nitroglycerin 0.4 mg SL up to three doses/alleviation of pain/or hypotension

5) Aspirin 325 mg

6) Consider morphine sulfate 2–5 mg IVP if BP does not drop from SL nitro

7) Rapid transport to appropriate facility

Detailed Physical Exam: En route to appropriate facility if time permits

Ongoing Assessment: There is no change in patient's condition during transport.

Critical Actions:
1) Secure airway and ensure highest oxygenation at 15 lpm via NRM; if respiratory failure, then PPV.

2) Maintain hemodynamic stability—BP between 70–100 mmHg, no higher

3) Attempt to reduce myocardial ischemia/necrosis.

Teaching Points

1) There are numerous causes and etiologies of chest pain. Assist the participant in classifying chest pain to body system and causes (e.g., cardiac vs. respiratory, trauma vs. medical) for rule outs.

2) Always follow an organized approach to rule out possible causes.

3) Compare and contrast clinical findings of an AMI to other presentations.

4) Compare and contrast the treatment of an AMI.

5) Review the indications of nitroglycerin, morphine, and aspirin in the management of this patient.

Evaluation

1) *Excellent:* The participant's evaluation of the patient followed set format: initial assessment, focused history (SAMPLE, OPQRST) in an efficient manner. The participant displayed a thorough knowledge of the patient's condition, performed the exam and management in an organized manner, and demonstrated an excellent overall performance.

2) *Good:* The participant's evaluation of the patient followed set format: initial assessment, focused history (SAMPLE, OPQRST) in an acceptable manner with only minor deviation. The participant displayed an above-average knowledge of the patient's condition, performed the

exam and management of the patient's condition, and demonstrated an above-average performance.

3) *Fair:* The participant's evaluation of the patient deviated from the set format without causing any further injury to the patient. The participant displayed an average or basic knowledge of the patient's condition and performed an adequate exam and management of the patient's condition.

4) *Inadequate:* The participant's evaluation of the patient deviated significantly from the set format, or the participant's actions endangered the patient's life or significantly exacerbated the condition.

▶ Chest Pain: Case 4

Requirements: One instructor and one patient for every five participants

Prerequisites: Read Chapter 4, "Hypoperfusion (Shock)" and Chapter 6, "Chest Pain."

Equipment: One table and chair for the patient to use; jump kit with oxygen supplies (NC, NRM, aerosol mask, PPV device, intubation equipment), stethoscope, BP cuff, cardiac monitor, pulse oximeter, and medication kit with associated medications

Instructor: Your role is vital as your must act as the coordinator of the station and also interact in the scenario. Before the participant arrives at the station, please review the scenario with your patient. Spray the patient's arms with a fine mist of cool water to simulate cool and clammy skin. Please read the scenario to become familiar with the necessary responses. Do not "coach" the participant along during the testing station; rather, allow him to conduct the exam without interruption or help.

Patient: One female (or male) patient. As the patient, you will be required to play the role of a 16-year-old female complaining of burning in your chest. You have suffered an esophageal disruption/tear from vomiting. Please read the scenario to familiarize yourself with the information. You will have a fine mist of water sprayed on you to simulate cool and diaphoretic skin.

Instructions

Hi, my name is _____ , and I will be the examiner for this station. This is a hands-on patient assessment station. You will be given information concerning a patient experiencing a medical crisis. You will have all the necessary equipment you need to manage the patient in this station. Please look over the equipment before we go any further. You will be provided with pertinent information only when you ask the appropriate question. For any hands-on procedure, such as auscultation of a blood pressure or breath sounds or taking a pulse, select the appropriate equipment needed (if any) and use the equipment in the manner that it would be used on a patient. I will then give you the relevant clinical data. For example, you must select, place, and begin inflation of the BP cuff before the blood pressure is given to you. I will not answer questions in place of the patient. Therefore, it is imperative that you interact with your patient. Please verbalize to me any signs or symptoms that you find so that I will know you are cognizant of the patient and the patient's clinical appearance.

Scenario

Advise the participant that he responding to a call of a 16-year-old female (or male) with chest pain. If the participant is a nurse or in-hospital provider, the scenario can be modified to the medical environment—such as someone rushes a 16-year-old patient in a wheelchair to your desk. The participant should use the assessment taught in this course.

Initial Impression: 16-year-old female (or male) lying on the bathroom floor (or sitting in a wheelchair) surrounded by vomitus and blood. The patient is awake, very anxious, appears cyanotic, and has accessory muscle usage.

Scene Size-up/General Impression: The scene is safe for entry and exit. No injury is apparent on brief visual exam.

Initial Assessment:

Mental Status—Responsive and alert to all commands

Airway—The patient has just finished vomiting.

Breathing—Respirations 36 and very shallow

Circulation—Radial pulse weak at 116 bpm, skin cool and diaphoretic

Disability—Moves all four extremities

Status after Initial Assessment: Critical, potentially life threatening.

Initial Management Priorities: High-flow oxygen at 15 lpm via NRM, cardiac monitor, IV access

Focused History (SAMPLE):

Signs and Symptoms—Chest pain, DIB, cool and diaphoretic skin

Allergies—NKA

Medications—None per patient

Past Medical History—None per patient

Last Oral Intake—Patient just finished eating.

Events Preceding—Patient states that she had just finished eating and felt sick to her stomach. She vomited once in the toilet and felt a tearing burning sensation in her chest. Then she felt dizzy and called her sister who called 911.

OPQRST:

Onset—Very sudden, right after I vomited.

Palliation/Provocation—Everything makes it burn worse.

Quality—It's a very sharp pain.

Radiation—In the middle of my chest and back.

Severity—It's the worst pain I've ever felt.

Time/Duration—Since whenever you were called

Vital Signs:

Respirations—36 and shallow

Pulse—Radial pulse irregular at 116 bpm and bounding

Blood Pressure—84/76

Temperature—98.5°F (37°C)

Pulse Oximetry—95%

Blood Glucose Level—112 mg/dl

Focused Physical Exam (Focused Medical Assessment): If the participant inquires about the vomiting, the sibling will reply, "I think she makes herself throw up after she eats."

Differential/Field Diagnosis: Esophageal disruption/tear

Management:

1) High-flow oxygen at 15 lpm via NRM

2) IV access—fluid bolus to maintain a systolic BP of 70–100 mmHg

3) Cardiac monitor

5) Transport

Detailed Physical Exam: En route to appropriate facility if time permits

Ongoing Assessment: There is no change in patient's condition during transport.

Critical Actions:

1) Secure airway and ensure highest oxygenation at 15 lpm via NRM; if respiratory failure, then PPV.

2) Maintain hemodynamic stability—BP between 70–100 mmHg, no higher.

Teaching Points

1) There are numerous causes and etiologies of chest pain. Assist the participant in classifying chest pain to body system and causes (e.g., cardiac vs. respiratory, trauma vs. medical) for rule outs.

2) Always follow an organized approach to rule out possible causes.

3) Compare and contrast clinical findings of an esophageal tear to other presentations.

4) Compare and contrast the treatment of an esophageal tear.

5) Review the management of this patient.

Evaluation

1) *Excellent:* The participant's evaluation of the patient followed set format: initial assessment, focused history (SAMPLE, OPQRST) in an efficient manner. The participant displayed a thorough knowledge of the patient's condition, performed the exam and management in an organized manner, and demonstrated an excellent overall performance.

2) *Good:* The participant's evaluation of the patient followed set format: initial assessment, focused history (SAMPLE, OPQRST) in an acceptable manner with only minor deviation. The participant displayed an above-average knowledge of the patient's condition, performed the exam and management of the patient's condition, and demonstrated an above-average performance.

3) *Fair:* The participant's evaluation of the patient deviated from the set format without causing any further injury to the patient. The participant displayed an average or basic knowledge of the patient's condition and performed an adequate exam and management of the patient's condition.

4) *Inadequate:* The participant's evaluation of the patient deviated significantly from the set format, or the participant's actions endangered the patient's life or significantly exacerbated the condition.

⊞ ALTERED MENTAL STATUS/SEIZURES AND SEIZURE DISORDERS

▶ ALTERED MENTAL STATUS/SEIZURES AND SEIZURE DISORDERS: CASE 1

Requirements: One instructor and one patient for every five participants

Prerequisites: Read Chapter 7, "Altered Mental Status" and Chapter 10, "Seizures and Seizure Disorders."

Equipment: One table and chair for the patient to use; jump kit with oxygen supplies (NC, NRM, acrosol mask, PPV device, intubation equipment), stethoscope, BP cuff, cardiac monitor, pulse oximeter, and medication kit with assorted medications

Instructor: Your role is vital as you must act as the coordinator of the station and also interact in the scenario. Before the participant arrives at the station, please review the scenario with your patient. For moulage, tint the patient's face with a blue coloring to simulate cyanosis. Then spray the patient's arms with a fine mist of cool water to simulate cool and clammy skin. Have the patient place a small amount of water in her mouth to help simulate "gurgling" respirations.

Patient: One female (or male) patient. As the patient, you will be required to play the role of a 34-year-old suffering from a decreased level of consciousness. Please breathe shallowly and at a slow rate—approximately 6 breaths per minute, if possible. Gurgle with each respiration until the participant suctions your mouth. You are completely unresponsive to verbal and painful stimuli. Please read the scenario to familiarize yourself with the information. You will have a fine mist of cold water sprayed onto your arms and face by the instructor to simulate cool and clammy skin.

Instructions

Hi, my name is _____ , and I will be the examiner for this station. This is a hands-on patient assessment station. You will be given information concerning a patient experiencing a medical crisis. You will have all the necessary equipment you need to manage the patient in this station. Please look over the equipment before we go any further. You will be provided with pertinent information only when you ask the appropriate question. For any hands-on procedure, such as auscultation of a blood pressure or breath sounds or taking a pulse, select the appropriate equipment needed (if any) and use the equipment in the manner that it would be used on a patient. I will then give you the relevant clinical data. For example, you must select, place, and begin inflation of the BP cuff before the blood pressure is given to you. I will not answer questions in place of the patient. Therefore, it is imperative that you interact with your patient. Please verbalize to me any signs or symptoms that you find so that I will know you are cognizant of the patient and the patient's clinical appearance.

Scenario

Advise the participant that she is responding to an unknown medical emergency. If the participant is a nurse or in-hospital provider, the scenario can be modified to the medical environment—such as reporting to triage after a shift change and park rangers have pulled up to the ED with a patient. The participant should use the assessment taught in this course.

Initial Impression: 34-year-old female (or male) lying supine on the park bench, unresponsive, with gurgling respirations

Scene Size-up/General Impression: Police are present and escort you to the patient. No weapons or evidence of drug or alcohol use are seen. No evidence of injury.

Initial Assessment:

Mental Status—AVPU: unresponsive to painful stimuli

Airway—Gurgling respirations indicating vomitus in mouth; C-spine precautions initiated.

Breathing—Respirations 6 and very shallow, unlabored

Circulation—Very slow and weak at 60 bpm, regular; skin cool, clammy, and pale, no external bleeding

Disability—Unable to move extremities with painful stimulation

Status after Initial Assessment: Life-threatening, unstable

Initial Management Priorities: Suction, oral or nasal airway device, cardiac monitor, blood glucose level, oxygen at 15 lpm with NRM, IV therapy, recovery position, prepare to intubate

Focused History (SAMPLE):

Signs and Symptoms—Unresponsive, peripheral cyanosis, cool and clammy skin

Allergies—Unknown

Medications—Unknown

Past Medical History—If the participant states he is looking for medical alert tags, the patient will have a tag with IDDM written on it.

Last Oral Intake—Unknown

Events Preceding—Per park rangers, the patient is a "regular" homeless inhabitant of the park. They found the patient on the park bench while on routine patrol.

OPQRST:

Onset—Unknown

Palliation/Provocation—Unknown

Quality—Unknown

Radiation—Unknown

Severity—Unknown

Time—One park ranger states that he saw the patient two hours before at the food shelter.

Vital Signs:

> *Respirations*—6 and shallow, unlabored (unless PPV was initiated)
>
> *Pulse*—Radial pulse 60 bpm and weak
>
> *Blood Pressure*—88/64
>
> *Temperature*—99.6°F (37.9°C)
>
> *Pulse Oximetry*—92%
>
> *Blood Glucose Level*—88 mg/dl

Focused Physical Exam (Focused Medical Assessment): Inspection shows the patient has multiple needle track marks on the anterior thighs, in the lower abdomen, and in the antecubital space; pupils are pinpoint and nonreactive.

Differential/Field Diagnosis: Unknown; unresponsive hypoglycemia versus drug overdose

Management:

1) Suction of oral pharynx

2) Insertion of oral pharyngeal airway (OPA) and/or nasopharyngeal airway (NPA)

3) PPV with supplemental oxygen

4) IV access—check blood glucose level (BGL)—88 mg/dl

5) Fluid bolus

6) Cardiac monitor—sinus bradycardia with no ectopy

7) Narcan 0.4–2.0 mg IVP

8) Thiamine 100 mg IVP/IM

9) Patient remains unresponsive—consider RSI:

   a) Defasciculating agent—vecuronium 0.01 mg/kg IVP

   b) Sedative—midazolam 0.05–0.1 mg/kg IVP, diazepam 0.2 mg/kg IVP, fentanyl 3–5 μg/kg, or any of the other sedatives

   c) Cricoid pressure

   d) Succinylcholine 1.5 mg/kg IVP

   e) Intubation

   f) Confirmation

Detailed Physical Exam: En route to appropriate facility if time permits

Ongoing Assessment: Every five minutes en route to appropriate facility

Critical Actions:

1) Suction and secure airway with endotracheal intubation to prevent aspiration.

2) Determine appropriate treatment modalities.

Teaching Points

1) There are numerous causes and etiologies of altered mental status.

2) Always follow an organized approach to rule out possible causes.

3) Don't let past medical history lead you to a diagnosis preemptively.

4) Discuss treatment priorities—suction and protect airway. Early intubation is not always warranted. Discuss why intubation may be deferred in the hypoglycemic and overdose patient until medical therapies, for example, dextrose (D_{50}) and Narcan, have been administered.

5) Explain the advantages and disadvantages of using an RSI.

6) Emphasize the need to no longer use the "coma cocktail" for all unknown unresponsive patients.

Evaluation

1) *Excellent:* The participant's evaluation of the patient followed set format: initial assessment, focused history (SAMPLE, OPQRST) in an efficient manner. The participant displayed a thorough knowledge of the patient's condition, performed the exam and management in an organized manner, and demonstrated an excellent overall performance.

2) *Good:* The participant's evaluation of the patient followed set format: initial assessment, focused history (SAMPLE, OPQRST) in an acceptable manner with only minor deviation. The participant displayed an above-average knowledge of the patient's condition, performed the exam and management of the patient's condition, and demonstrated an above-average performance.

3) *Fair:* The participant's evaluation of the patient deviated from the set format without causing any further injury to the patient. The participant displayed an average or basic knowledge of the patient's condition and performed an adequate exam and management of the patient's condition.

4) *Inadequate:* The participant's evaluation of the patient deviated significantly from the set format, or the participant's actions endangered the patient's life or significantly exacerbated the condition.

▶ ALTERED MENTAL STATUS/SEIZURES AND SEIZURE DISORDERS: CASE 2

Requirements: One instructor and one patient for every five participants

Prerequisites: Read Chapter 7, "Altered Mental Status" and Chapter 10, "Seizures and Seizure Disorders."

Equipment: One table and chair for the patient to use; jump kit with oxygen supplies (NC, NRM, aerosol mask, PPV device, intubation equipment), stethoscope, BP cuff, cardiac monitor, pulse oximeter, and medication kit with assorted medications

Instructor: Your role is vital as you must act as the coordinator of the station and also interact in the scenario. Before the participant arrives at the station, please review the scenario with your patient. Spray the patient's arms with a fine mist of cool water to simulate cool and clammy skin. For moulage, tint the patient's face with a blue coloring to simulate cyanosis. Have the patient place an artificial blood pill in his mouth. Instruct the patient to break the pill, allowing blood to trickle out of his mouth. You will act as the patient's friend and answer the questions as best as you can.

Patient: One male (or female) patient. As the patient, you will be required to play the role of a 24-year-old male suffering from a generalized tonic-clonic seizure. Please move your arms and legs, rhythmically interrupted by a short period of "stiffness" of the extremities. You will not respond to any verbal or painful stimuli. Please read the scenario to familiarize yourself with the information.

Instructions

Hi, my name is _____ , and I will be the examiner for this station. This is a hands-on patient assessment station. You will be given information concerning a patient experiencing a medical crisis. You will have all the necessary equipment you need to manage the patient in this station. Please look over the equipment before we go any further. You will be provided with pertinent information only when you ask the appropriate question. For any hands-on procedure, such as auscultation of a blood pressure or breath sounds or taking a pulse, select the appropriate equipment needed (if any) and use the equipment in the manner that it would be used on a patient. I will then give you the relevant clinical data. For example, you must select, place, and begin inflation of the BP cuff before the blood pressure is given to you. I will not answer questions in place of the patient. Therefore, it is imperative that you interact with your patient. Please verbalize to me any signs or symptoms that you find so that I will know you are cognizant of the patient and the patient's clinical appearance.

Scenario

Advise the participant that he is responding to a possible seizure in the grocery store. If the participant is a nurse or in-hospital provider, the scenario can be modified to the medical environment—such as reporting to triage after a shift change where a patient is lying on the floor apparently having a seizure. The participant should use the assessment taught in this course.

Initial Impression: 24-year-old male (or female) lying supine on the floor flailing around, apparently having a seizure

Scene Size-up/General Impression: The store manager escorts you to the patient. Store employees have shoppers under control. Police department has been notified of incident and is responding.

Initial Assessment:

Mental Status—AVPU: unresponsive to verbal commands

Airway—Blood coming out of the mouth

Breathing—Respirations 40 and very shallow

Circulation—Present, but difficult to assess because of seizure activity; no evidence of injury, no external bleeding

Disability—Tonic-clonic movement

Status after Initial Assessment: Life-threatening, unstable

Initial Management Priorities: Oxygen at 15 lpm NRM, recovery position, suction. When accessible: IV therapy, blood glucose level, pulse oximetry, cardiac monitor. Management is focused on safety of patient initially. Secondary management when accessible is to stop the seizure and determine the underlying cause. Prepare to insert oral or nasal airway and intubate if necessary.

Focused History (SAMPLE):

Signs and Symptoms—Unresponsive, peripheral cyanosis, cool and clammy skin

Allergies—Friend doesn't know.

Medications—Some sort of medicine to stop the "fits"

Past Medical History—Per friend, the "fits" started a year ago after a car accident.

Last Oral Intake—Approximately 30 minutes ago, beer and chips

Events Preceding—The friend states that the patient had been drinking beer all day while watching movies. They ran out of beer and decided to go to the grocery store to pick some more up.

OPQRST:

Onset—It started about 3 minutes ago. Moves all extremities in a tonic-clonic fashion

Palliation/Provocation—The patient told his friend that the lights were bothering his eyes.

Quality—Tonic-clonic movement

Radiation—All four extremities

Severity—Tonic-clonic movement

Time—Per friend, the "fit" came on suddenly as they were walking down the aisle. Seizure has been going on for 10 minutes.

Vital Signs:

> *Respirations*—40 and very shallow (unless PPV was initiated)
>
> *Pulse*—Radial pulse rapid, 130 bpm, regular
>
> *Blood Pressure*—Unobtainable
>
> *Temperature*—Unobtainable
>
> *Pulse Oximetry*—Unobtainable

Focused Physical Exam (Focused Medical Assessment): Patient continues to have tonic-clonic movement; stain in pants indicates patient lost bowel control; blood from mouth indicates possible tongue laceration.

Differential/Field Diagnoses: Acute generalized seizure

Management:

1) C-spine control

2) Suction of oral pharynx, if possible

3) Insertion of OPA and/or NPA

4) Supplemental oxygen at 15 lpm via NRM

5) IV access—check BGL—88 mg/dl

6) Cardiac monitor, when obtainable—sinus tachycardia with no ectopy

7) Diazepam 2–10 mg IVP

(Seizure activity does stop and patient is postictal.)

Detailed Physical Exam: En route to appropriate facility if time permits

Ongoing Assessment: Every 5 minutes while en route to the receiving facility

Critical Actions:

1) Suction and secure airway, insert OPA or NPA.

2) Stop the seizure activity.

Teaching Points

1) There are numerous causes and etiologies of seizures.

2) Always follow an organized approach to rule out possible causes.

3) Don't let past medical history lead you to a diagnosis preemptively.

4) Discuss treatment priorities—suction and protect airway. Early intubation is not always warranted. Highest priority is to stop the seizure activity.

5) Discuss how valium can be administered if IV access is not possible due to seizure activity.

Evaluation

1) *Excellent:* The participant's evaluation of the patient followed set format: initial assessment, focused history (SAMPLE, OPQRST) in an efficient manner. The participant displayed a thorough knowledge of the patient's condition, performed the exam and management in an organized manner, and demonstrated an excellent overall performance.

2) *Good:* The participant's evaluation of the patient followed set format: initial assessment, focused history (SAMPLE, OPQRST) in an acceptable manner with only minor deviation. The participant displayed an above-average knowledge of the patient's condition, performed the exam and management of the patient's condition, and demonstrated an above-average performance.

3) *Fair:* The participant's evaluation of the patient deviated from the set format without causing any further injury to the patient. The participant displayed an average or basic knowledge of the patient's condition and performed an adequate exam and management of the patient's condition.

4) *Inadequate:* The participant's evaluation of the patient deviated significantly from the set format, or the participant's actions endangered the patient's life or significantly exacerbated the condition.

► ALTERED MENTAL STATUS/SEIZURES AND SEIZURE DISORDERS: CASE 3

Requirements: One instructor and one patient for every five participants

Prerequisites: Read Chapter 7, "Altered Mental Status" and Chapter 10, "Seizures and Seizure Disorders."

Equipment: One table and chair for the patient to use; jump kit with oxygen supplies (NC, NRM, aerosol mask, PPV device, intubation equipment), stethoscope, BP cuff, cardiac monitor, pulse oximeter, and medication kit with assorted medications

Instructor: Your role is vital as you must act as the coordinator of the station and also interact in the scenario. Before the participant arrives at the station, please review the scenario with your patient. Spray the patient's arms with a fine mist of cool water to simulate cool and clammy skin. For moulage, tint the patient's face with a blue coloring to simulate cyanosis.

Patient: One female (or male) patient. As the patient, you will be required to play the role of a 22-year-old female suffering from a decreased level of consciousness. You will be unresponsive to verbal stimuli and moan when deep painful stimuli is performed. Place a small amount of liquid in your mouth to simulate gurgling respirations. Please read the scenario to familiarize yourself with the information.

Instructions

Hi, my name is _____ , and I will be the examiner for this station. This is a hands-on patient assessment station. You will be given information concerning a patient experiencing a medical crisis. You will have all the necessary equipment you need to manage the patient in this station. Please look over the equipment before we go any further. You will be provided with pertinent information only when you ask the appropriate question. For any hands-on procedure, such as auscultation of a blood pressure or breath sounds or taking a pulse, select the appropriate equipment needed (if any) and use the equipment in the manner that it would be used on a patient. I will then give you the relevant clinical data. For example, you must select, place, and begin inflation of the BP cuff before the blood pressure is given to you. I will not answer questions in place of the patient. Therefore, it is imperative that you interact with your patient. Please verbalize to me any signs or symptoms that you find so that I will know you are cognizant of the patient and the patient's clinical appearance.

Scenario

Advise the participant that she is responding to a possible overdose. On the scene is a friend who found the patient lying on the bathroom floor with the medicine cabinet open. If the participant is a nurse or in-hospital provider, the scenario can be modified to the medical environment—such as reporting to triage after a shift change where a hysterical friend drags the patient into the ED. The participant should use the assessment taught in this course.

Initial Impression: 24-year-old female (or male) lying supine on the floor, unresponsive, with gurgling respirations

Scene Size-up/General Impression: There is easy access in and out of the residence. Patient's friend escorts you to patient lying on bathroom floor.

Initial Assessment:

Mental Status—AVPU: unresponsive to verbal commands, moans to deep painful stimuli

Airway—Small amount of saliva in oral pharynx

Breathing—Respirations 8 and very shallow, unlabored

Circulation—Radial pulse weak and thready at 64 bpm, irregular; there is no evidence of injury or bleeding.

Disability—No response to painful stimuli

Status after Initial Assessment: Life-threatening, unstable

Initial Management Priorities: Airway maintenance with nasal or oral airway device, oxygen at 15 lpm via NRM, pulse oximetry, IV therapy, monitor, recovery position, prepare to intubate

Focused History (SAMPLE):

Signs and Symptoms—Unresponsive, peripheral cyanosis, cool and clammy skin

Allergies—Friend doesn't know.

Medications—In the medicine cabinet are over-the-counter (OTC) analgesic and sinus medications along with TB syringes and alcohol pads.

Past Medical History—Per friend, the patient is very reclusive and she is unaware of any.

Last Oral Intake—Per friend, this morning at breakfast

Events Preceding—The friend states that they had met this morning for breakfast at the mall. The patient looked ill and wasn't feeling well. Consequently, she didn't eat anything and went home to "sleep off her headache."

OPQRST:

Onset—Unknown

Palliation/Provocation—Unknown

Quality—Unknown

Radiation—Unknown

Severity—Unknown

Time—Unknown

Vital Signs:

Respirations—8 and shallow (unless PPV was initiated)

Pulse—Radial pulse weak and thready at 128 bpm

Blood Pressure—118/76

Temperature—98.2°F (36.8°C)

Pulse Oximetry—93%

Blood Glucose Level—48 mg/dl

Focused Physical Exam (Focused Medical Assessment): Patient remains responsive only to deep painful stimuli; pupils equal and reactive to light, but a little slow to react. No bruising or injury noted. No medical alert identification found.

Differential/Field Diagnosis: Unknown unresponsive with hypoglycemic episode

Management:

1) C-spine control

2) Suction of oral pharynx, if possible

3) Insertion of OPA and/or NPA

4) PPV ventilation with supplemental oxygen

5) IV access—check BGL—48 mg/dl

6) Dextrose (D_{50}) 25 grams slow IVP—glucagon 1 mg IM if IV unobtainable

7) Cardiac monitor—sinus tachycardia with occasional PACs

Detailed Physical Exam: En route to appropriate facility if time permits

Ongoing Assessment: Every 5 minutes while en route to the receiving facility

Critical Actions:

1) Suction and secure airway, insert OPA or NPA.

2) Check BGL and pupils to determine possible causes.

Teaching Points

1) There are numerous causes and etiologies of an unknown unresponsive.

2) Always follow an organized approach to rule out possible causes.

3) Don't let scene clues lead you to a diagnosis preemptively. (The patient could have been trying to get some sugar candies out of the medicine cabinet when she collapsed.)

4) Discuss treatment priorities—suction and protect airway. Early intubation is not always warranted. Highest priority is to provide glucose to the body.

Evaluation

1) *Excellent:* The participant's evaluation of the patient followed set format: initial assessment, focused history (SAMPLE, OPQRST) in an efficient manner. The participant displayed a thorough knowledge of the patient's condition, performed the exam and management in an organized manner, and demonstrated an excellent overall performance.

2) *Good:* The participant's evaluation of the patient followed set format: initial assessment, focused history (SAMPLE, OPQRST) in an acceptable manner with only minor deviation. The participant displayed an

above-average knowledge of the patient's condition, performed the exam and management of the patient's condition, and demonstrated an above-average performance.

3) *Fair:* The participant's evaluation of the patient deviated from the set format without causing any further injury to the patient. The participant displayed an average or basic knowledge of the patient's condition and performed an adequate exam and management of the patient's condition.

4) *Inadequate:* The participant's evaluation of the patient deviated significantly from the set format, or the participant's actions endangered the patient's life or significantly exacerbated the condition.

▶ ALTERED MENTAL STATUS/SEIZURES AND SEIZURE DISORDERS: CASE 4

Requirements: One instructor and one patient for every five participants

Prerequisites: Read Chapter 7, "Altered Mental Status" and Chapter 10, "Seizures and Seizure Disorders."

Equipment: One table and chair for the patient to use; jump kit with oxygen supplies (NC, NRM, aerosol mask, PPV device, intubation equipment), stethoscope, BP cuff, cardiac monitor, pulse oximeter, and medication kit with assorted medications

Instructor: Your role is vital as you must act as the coordinator of the station and also interact in the scenario. Before the participant arrives at the station, please review the scenario with your patient. Spray the patient's arms with a fine mist of cool water to simulate cool and clammy skin. You will act as the patient's spouse and answer all questions.

Patient: One male (or female) patient. As the patient, you will be required to play the role of a 32-year-old male suffering from an acute decreased level of consciousness. You will be unresponsive to verbal stimuli and moan when deep painful stimuli is performed. Please breathe at a very fast and shallow rate, approximately 40 times per minute. Please read the scenario to familiarize yourself with the information.

Instructions

Hi, my name is _____ , and I will be the examiner for this station. This is a hands-on patient assessment station. You will be given information concerning a patient experiencing a medical crisis. You will have all the necessary equipment you need to manage the patient in this station. Please look over the equipment before we go any further. You will be provided with pertinent information only when you ask the appropriate question. For any hands-on procedure, such as auscultation of a blood pressure or breath sounds or taking a pulse, select the appropriate equipment needed (if any) and use the equipment in the manner that it would be used on a patient. I will then give you the relevant clinical data. For example, you must select, place, and begin inflation of the BP cuff before the blood pressure is given to you. I will not answer questions in place of the patient. Therefore, it is imperative that you interact with your patient. Please verbalize to me any signs or symptoms that you find so that I will know you are cognizant of the patient and the patient's clinical appearance.

Scenario

Advise the participant that he is responding to a "man down" call. He arrives on scene to find the patient on the floor in the bedroom. If the participant is a nurse or in-hospital provider, the scenario can be modified to the medical environment—such as reporting to triage after a shift change where an anxious wife has run into the waiting room asking for help to get her spouse out of the car. The participant should use the assessment taught in this course.

Initial Impression: 32-year-old male (or female) lying supine on the floor

Scene Size-up/General Impression: Neighbor lets you access the home from the front door. There is easy access in and out of the residence. There are no animals or appearance of violence.

Initial Assessment:

Mental Status—AVPU: unresponsive to verbal commands, moans to deep painful stimuli; no injury apparent

Airway—Clear and patent at this time

Breathing—Respirations 40 and very shallow, unlabored

Circulation—Radial pulse weak and thready at 114 bpm, no external bleeding present

Disability—Distal pulses thready

Status after Initial Assessment: Life-threatening, unstable

Initial Management Priorities: Airway maintenance with oral or nasal airway, oxygen at 15 lpm via NRM, pulse oximetry, cardiac monitor, IV therapy, blood glucose level, suction if necessary

Focused History (SAMPLE):

Signs and Symptoms—Unresponsive with rapid respirations

Allergies—Spouse states none.

Medications—Adalat

Past Medical History—Significant for hypertension

Last Oral Intake—This morning at breakfast

Events Preceding—The spouse states that they had just finished having sexual intercourse when the patient got out of bed to use the bathroom. He complained of a "killer headache, the worst he ever had" and then suddenly collapsed on the floor.

OPQRST:

Onset—Rapid

Palliation/Provocation—Unknown

Quality—Unknown

Radiation—Spouse states that the patient had said the pain was just in his head.

Severity—"Killer headache, the worst of his life"

Time—Approximately 10 minutes ago

Vital Signs:

Respirations—40 and very shallow (unless PPV was initiated)

Pulse—Radial pulse weak and thready at 114 bpm

Blood Pressure—214/168

Temperature—98.2°F (36.8°C)

Pulse Oximetry—90%

Blood Glucose Level—112 mg/dl

Focused Physical Exam (Focused Medical Assessment): Patient remains responsive only to deep painful stimuli; right pupil is dilated and non-reactive. No signs of injury present.

Differential/Field Diagnosis: Unknown unresponsive, possible hemorrhagic bleed

Management:

1) Insertion of OPA and/or NPA

2) PPV ventilation with supplemental oxygen

3) IV access

4) Cardiac monitor—sinus tachycardia with no ectopy

5) Endotracheal intubation via RSI

    a) Defasciculating agent—vecuronium 0.01 mg/kg IVP

    b) Sedative—midazolam 0.05–0.1 mg/kg IVP, diazepam 0.2 mg/kg IVP, fentanyl 3–5 µg/kg, or any of the other sedatives

    c) Cricoid pressure

    d) Succinylcholine 1.5 mg/kg IVP

    e) Intubation

    f) Confirmation

6) Positive pressure ventilation to help decrease intracranial pressure

7) Rapid transport to appropriate facility

Detailed Physical Exam: En route to appropriate facility if time permits

Ongoing Assessment: En route to the receiving facility every 5 minutes

Critical Actions:

1) PPV with supplemental oxygen

2) Endotracheal intubation with RSI to secure the airway and provide hyperventilation

3) Do not treat with hypertonic or dextrose solutions.

4) DO NOT TREAT THE ELEVATED BLOOD PRESSURE.

Teaching Points

1) There are numerous causes and etiologies of an unknown unresponsive.

2) Always follow an organized approach to rule out possible causes.

3) Don't let scene clues lead you to a diagnosis preemptively. (As humorous as the scene may have initially appeared, the outcome was deadly.)

4) Discuss treatment priorities—PPV with supplemental oxygen and RSI.

5) Discuss the effects of dextrose and hypertonic solutions.

6) Discuss the effects of lowering the blood pressure.

Evaluation

1) *Excellent:* The participant's evaluation of the patient followed set format: initial assessment, focused history (SAMPLE, OPQRST) in an efficient manner. The participant displayed a thorough knowledge of the patient's condition, performed the exam and management in an organized manner, and demonstrated an excellent overall performance.

2) *Good:* The participant's evaluation of the patient followed set format: initial assessment, focused history (SAMPLE, OPQRST) in an acceptable manner with only minor deviation. The participant displayed an above-average knowledge of the patient's condition, performed the exam and management of the patient's condition, and demonstrated an above-average performance.

3) *Fair:* The participant's evaluation of the patient deviated from the set format without causing any further injury to the patient. The participant displayed an average or basic knowledge of the patient's condition and performed an adequate exam and management of the patient's condition.

4) *Inadequate:* The participant's evaluation of the patient deviated significantly from the set format, or the participant's actions endangered the patient's life or significantly exacerbated the condition.

▦ ACUTE ABDOMINAL PAIN/GI BLEEDING

▶ ACUTE ABDOMINAL PAIN/GI BLEEDING: CASE 1

Requirements: One instructor and one patient for every five participants

Prerequisites: Read Chapter 8, "Acute Abdominal Pain"; Chapter 9, "Gastrointestinal Bleeding"; and Chapter 12, "Headache, Nausea, and Vomiting."

Equipment: One table and chair for the patient to use; jump kit with oxygen supplies (NC, NRM, aerosol mask, PPV device, intubation equipment), stethoscope, BP cuff, cardiac monitor, pulse oximeter, and medication kit with associated medications

Instructor: Your role is vital as your must act as the coordinator of the station and also interact in the scenario. Before the participant arrives at the station, please review the scenario with your patient. For moulage, tint the patient's anterior abdomen and lower extremities with a blue coloring to simulate cyanosis. Please read the scenario to become familiar with the necessary responses. Do not "coach" the participant along during the testing station; rather, allow him to conduct the exam without interruption or help.

Patient: One female (or male) patient. As the patient, you will be required to play the role of a 60-year-old female suffering from acute abdominal pain. You are awake and alert and can answer all questions. The pain started right after breakfast this morning. The pain is a "steady pain" in the mid-abdominal area that moves to the back. Your medical history includes hypertension, for which you take Aldactazide, and non-insulin-dependent diabetes mellitus (NIDDM), for which you take Glucophage. You are lying supine on the couch, which greatly decreases the pain. Please read the scenario to familiarize yourself with the information.

Instructions

Hi, my name is _____ , and I will be the examiner for this station. This is a hands-on patient assessment station. You will be given information concerning a patient experiencing a medical crisis. You will have all the necessary equipment you need to manage the patient in this station. Please look over the equipment before we go any further. You will be provided with pertinent information only when you ask the appropriate question. For any hands-on procedure, such as auscultation of a blood pressure or breath sounds or taking a pulse, select the appropriate equipment needed (if any) and use the equipment in the manner that it would be used on a patient. I will then give you the relevant clinical data. For example, you must select, place, and begin inflation of the BP cuff before the blood pressure is given to you. I will not answer questions in place of the patient. Therefore, it is imperative that you interact with your patient. Please verbalize to me any signs or symptoms that you find so that I will know you are cognizant of the patient and the patient's clinical appearance.

Scenario

Advise the participant that she is responding to a call of abdominal pain. If the participant is a nurse or in-hospital provider, the scenario can be modified to the medical environment—such as a van has pulled up and the spouse has come into the ED to get you. The participant should use the assessment taught in this course.

Initial Impression: 60-year-old female (or male) lying supine on the couch, complaining of abdominal pain

Scene Size-up/General Impression: The scene is safe for entry and exit. No injury is apparent on brief visual exam. Family escorts you to the patient.

Initial Assessment:

Mental Status—Responsive, A&O × 3

Airway—Open and patent.

Breathing—Respirations 18 and regular, breath sounds equal and clear bilateral.

Circulation—Radial pulse 90 and regular, skin cool and dry.

Disability—Obeys all commands

Status after Initial Assessment: Serious, no immediate intervention needed at this time

Initial Management Priorities: Oxygen at 15 lpm via NRM, cardiac monitor, IV access

Focused History (SAMPLE):

Signs and Symptoms—Abdominal pain

Allergies—NKA

Medications—Aldactazide and Glucophage

Past Medical History—Hypertension and NIDDM; the patient might have forgotten to take her medication.

Last Oral Intake—Last night; at breakfast the patient wasn't feeling well enough to eat.

Events Preceding—This morning the patient didn't feel well and had vague abdominal pain, which has gotten worse.

OPQRST:

Onset—It was right before breakfast this morning at 9:00 A.M.

Palliation/Provocation—When I lie down, it feels much better.

Quality—At first it was vague, now it's a steady pain.

Radiation—It goes to my back, making it ache.

Severity—On a scale of 1 to 10, it's a 6.

Time/Duration—It's been a steady pain for about 2 hours now.

Vital Signs:

Respirations—18 and regular

Pulse—Radial pulse 90 bpm and regular

Blood Pressure—110/78

Temperature—99.6°F (37.9°C)

Pulse Oximetry—94% if on upper extremities; on lower extremities it won't measure.

Blood Glucose Level—120 mg/dl

Focused Physical Exam (Focused Medical Assessment): Rapid head-to-toe, patient's abdomen and lower extremities ashen and mottled. She has weak distal (dorsal pedis) pulses. Palpation reveals her abdomen is distended and tender.

Differential/Field Diagnosis: Possible abdominal aortic aneurysm (AAA).

Management:

1) High-flow oxygen at 15 lpm via NRM

2) Do not have the patient stand or walk to cot. Place patient is position of comfort.

3) Rapid transport to a hospital with surgical capabilities.

4) Establish 2 large-bore IVs en route running at a TKO rate unless patient is hypotensive.

5) Cardiac monitor—normal sinus rhythm with no ectopy

Detailed Physical Exam: En route to appropriate facility if time permits

Ongoing Assessment: Continue to monitor respiratory and cardiovascular status. Maintain position of comfort.

Critical Actions:

1) Utilize assessment clues of mottled lower extremities and weak lower peripheral pulses, along with the description of pain to come to the field diagnosis of acute abdominal aneurysm.

2) Recognize the potential for an unstable situation.

3) Transport gently and rapidly.

Teaching Points

1) There are numerous causes and etiologies of abdominal pain. Assist the participant in classifying abdominal pain to body system and causes (e.g., cardiovascular vs. gastrointestinal, trauma vs. medical) for rule outs.

2) Always follow an organized approach to rule out possible causes.

3) Don't let past medical history lead you to a diagnosis preemptively.

4) Discuss treatment priorities emphasizing the need for surgery. Emphasize that palpation should be gentle and done only once. Intravenous fluid therapy should be kept at a TKO rate unless the patient becomes hemodynamically unstable.

Evaluation

1) *Excellent:* The participant's evaluation of the patient followed set format: initial assessment, focused history (SAMPLE, OPQRST) in an efficient manner. The participant displayed a thorough knowledge of the patient's condition, performed the exam and management in an organized manner, and demonstrated an excellent overall performance.

2) *Good:* The participant's evaluation of the patient followed set format: initial assessment, focused history (SAMPLE, OPQRST) in an acceptable manner with only minor deviation. The participant displayed an above-average knowledge of the patient's condition, performed the exam and management of the patient's condition, and demonstrated an above-average performance.

3) *Fair:* The participant's evaluation of the patient deviated from the set format without causing any further injury to the patient. The participant displayed an average or basic knowledge of the patient's condition and performed an adequate exam and management of the patient's condition.

4) *Inadequate:* The participant's evaluation of the patient deviated significantly from the set format, or the participant's actions endangered the patient's life or significantly exacerbated the condition.

▶ ACUTE ABDOMINAL PAIN/GI BLEEDING: CASE 2

> **Requirements:** One instructor and one patient for every five participants
>
> **Prerequisites:** Read Chapter 8, "Acute Abdominal Pain"; Chapter 9, "Gastrointestinal Bleeding"; and Chapter 12, "Headache, Nausea, and Vomiting."
>
> **Equipment:** One table and chair for the patient to use; jump kit with oxygen supplies (NC, NRM, aerosol mask, PPV device, intubation equipment), stethoscope, BP cuff, cardiac monitor, pulse oximeter, and medication kit with associated medications

Instructor: Your role is vital as your must act as the coordinator of the station and also interact in the scenario. Before the participant arrives at the station, please review the scenario with your patient. Spray the patient's arms with a fine mist of cool water to simulate cool and clammy skin. For moulage, tint the patient's arms with a blue coloring to simulate cyanosis. Have the patient place an artificial blood capsule in his mouth and instruct him to break the pill and allow blood to trickle out of his mouth. Do not "coach" the participant along during the testing station; rather, allow him to conduct the exam without interruption or help.

Patient: One male (or female) patient. As the patient, you will be required to play the role of a 34-year-old male suffering from abdominal pain with bloody emesis. Please read the scenario to familiarize yourself with the information.

Instructions

Hi, my name is _____ , and I will be the examiner for this station. This is a hands-on patient assessment station. You will be given information concerning a patient experiencing a medical crisis. You will have all the necessary equipment you need to manage the patient in this station. Please look over the equipment before we go any further. You will be provided with pertinent information only when you ask the appropriate question. For any hands-on procedure, such as auscultation of a blood pressure or breath sounds or taking a pulse, select the appropriate equipment needed (if any) and use the equipment in the manner that it would be used on a patient. I will then give you the relevant clinical data. For example, you must select, place, and begin inflation of the BP cuff before the blood pressure is given to you. I will not answer questions in place of the patient. Therefore, it is imperative that you interact with your patient. Please verbalize to me any signs or symptoms that you find so that I will know you are cognizant of the patient and the patient's clinical appearance.

Scenario

Advise the participant that he is responding to an abdominal pain call. If the participant is a nurse or in-hospital provider, the scenario can be modified to the medical environment—such as the patient walked into the ED and collapsed in the triage seat. The participant should use the assessment taught in this course.

Initial Impression: 34-year-old male (or female) sitting in a chair, doubled over complaining of an intense burning in his stomach.

Scene Size-up/General Impression: The scene is safe for entry and exit. No injury is apparent on brief visual exam, although patient has blood around mouth.

Initial Assessment:

Mental Status—Responsive to all commands

Airway—Clear at this moment, but the patient does have bouts of emesis

Breathing—Respirations 26 and very shallow

Circulation—Radial pulse weak and thready, barely palpable

Disability—Moves all four extremities

Status after Initial Assessment: Immediate life threat

Initial Management Priorities: Oxygen at 15 lpm via NRM, cardiac monitor, IV access, position of comfort

Focused History (SAMPLE):

Signs and Symptoms—Responsive, peripheral cyanosis, cool and clammy skin

Allergies—NKA

Medications—An aspirin a day to prevent another MI

Past Medical History—History of an MI 3 years ago

Last Oral Intake—Approximately 6 1/2 hours ago, beer and chips

Events Preceding—Patient stated that he went out last night and had a few drinks, and the pain started about 2 hours after.

OPQRST:

Onset—It started slowly about 6 hours ago.

Palliation/Provocation—It's worse when I vomit.

Quality—It's a burning pain.

Radiation—It goes from my stomach all the way up and through my mouth.

Severity—It's a lot worse (burning sensation) when I vomit.

Time/Duration—It got worse approximately 2 hours ago.

Vital Signs:

Respirations—26 and shallow

Pulse—Radial pulse rapid and weak

Blood Pressure—64/palpation

Temperature—98.8°F (37°C)

Pulse Oximetry—94%

Blood Glucose Level—107 mg/dl

Focused Physical Exam (Focused Medical Assessment): Patient appears to have increasing pain; the vomitus appears to be brown in color and clumped (hematemesis).

Differential/Field Diagnosis: Acute GI bleed/hypoperfusion

Management:

1) Supplemental oxygen at 15 lpm via NRM

2) IV access × 2, large bore (14–16 gauge) with 250–500 cc fluid bolus to maintain a systolic BP between 70–100 mmHg

3) Cardiac monitor

4) Transport

Detailed Physical Exam: En route to appropriate facility if time permits

Ongoing Assessment: There is no change in patient's condition during transport.

Critical Actions:

1) Secure airway and ensure highest oxygenation at 15 lpm via NRM.

2) Maintain hemodynamic stability—BP between 70–100 mmHg, no higher.

Teaching Points

1) There are numerous causes and etiologies of abdominal pain. Assist the participant in classifying abdominal pain to body system and causes (e.g., cardiovascular vs. gastrointestinal, trauma vs. medical) for rule outs.

2) Always follow an organized approach to rule out possible causes.

3) Past medical history and current medications (aspirin) help with diagnosis.

4) Treatment priorities are to maintain oxygenation and hemodynamic stability.

Evaluation

1) *Excellent:* The participant's evaluation of the patient followed set format: initial assessment, focused history (SAMPLE, OPQRST) in an efficient manner. The participant displayed a thorough knowledge of the patient's condition, performed the exam and management in an organized manner, and demonstrated an excellent overall performance.

2) *Good:* The participant's evaluation of the patient followed set format: initial assessment, focused history (SAMPLE, OPQRST) in an acceptable manner with only minor deviation. The participant displayed an above-average knowledge of the patient's condition, performed the exam and management of the patient's condition, and demonstrated an above-average performance.

3) *Fair:* The participant's evaluation of the patient deviated from the set format without causing any further injury to the patient. The participant displayed an average or basic knowledge of the patient's condition and performed an adequate exam and management of the patient's condition.

4) *Inadequate:* The participant's evaluation of the patient deviated significantly from the set format, or the participant's actions endangered the patient's life or significantly exacerbated the condition.

► ACUTE ABDOMINAL PAIN/GI BLEEDING: CASE 3

Requirements: One instructor and one patient for every five participants

Prerequisites: Read Chapter 8 "Acute Abdominal Pain"; Chapter 9 "Gastrointestinal Bleeding"; and Chapter 12 "Headache, Nausea, and Vomiting."

Equipment: One table and chair for the patient to use; jump kit with oxygen supplies (NC, NRM, aerosol mask, PPV device, intubation equipment), stethoscope, BP cuff, cardiac monitor, pulse oximeter, and medication kit with associated medications

Instructor: Your role is vital as your must act as the coordinator of the station and also interact in the scenario. Before the participant arrives at the station, please review the scenario with your patient. Spray the patient's arms with a fine mist of cool water to simulate cool and clammy skin. Please read the scenario to become familiar with the necessary responses. Do not "coach" the participant along during the testing station; rather, allow him to conduct the exam without interruption or help.

Patient: One female (or male) patient. As the patient, you will be required to play the role of a 56-year-old female suffering from acute abdominal pain. You will be responsive and answer all questions. Please read the scenario to familiarize yourself with the information. You will have a fine mist of water sprayed on you to simulate cool and diaphoretic skin.

Instructions

Hi, my name is _____ , and I will be the examiner for this station. This is a hands-on patient assessment station. You will be given information concerning a patient experiencing a medical crisis. You will have all the necessary equipment you need to manage the patient in this station. Please look over the equipment before we go any further. You will be provided with pertinent information only when you ask the appropriate question. For any hands-on procedure, such as auscultation of a blood pressure or breath sounds or taking a pulse, select the appropriate equipment needed (if any) and use the equipment in the manner that it would be used on a patient. I will then give you the relevant clinical data. For example, you must select, place, and begin inflation of the BP cuff before the blood pressure is given to you. I will not answer questions in place of the patient. Therefore, it is imperative that you interact with your patient. Please verbalize to me any signs or symptoms that you find so that I will know you are cognizant of the patient and the patient's clinical appearance.

Scenario

Advise the participant that she is responding to an abdominal pain call. If the participant is a nurse or in-hospital provider, the scenario can be modified to the medical environment—such as the triage nurse brings a patient who complains of "abdominal pain" to Medical Room 1. The participant should use the assessment taught in this course.

Initial Impression: 56-year-old female (or male) lying on the floor/bed in the fetal position

Scene Size-up/General Impression: The scene is safe for entry and exit. No injury is apparent on brief visual exam. At the scene, the patient is lying on the floor near the telephone.

Initial Assessment:

Mental Status—Responsive and alert to all commands

Airway—Clear and patent at this time, but you notice a large amount of vomitus in a bucket

Breathing—Respirations 32 and very shallow

Circulation—Radial pulse bounding at 112 bpm

Disability—Barely moves all four extremities, but is reluctant to move due to movement causing pain

Status after Initial Assessment: Stable, potentially serious

Initial Management Priorities: Oxygen therapy as tolerated by patient, cardiac monitor, IV access

Focused History (SAMPLE):

Signs and Symptoms—Lying in the fetal position, shallow respirations, cool and clammy skin

Allergies—Tagamet and amoxicillin

Medications—Unknown sinus medication

Past Medical History—Intermittent abdominal pain for past year but it always went away so the patient never had it "checked out."

Last Oral Intake—Nothing since that "all you can eat" fish dinner last night.

Events Preceding—After the patient arrived home last night, she developed abdominal pain. She spent most of the night pacing back and forth around the house, which alleviated the pain. Then the pain got so extreme that she was unable to walk and lay on the bed in the fetal position.

OPQRST:

Onset—It started suddenly last night after dinner.

Palliation/Provocation—At first walking around, now just lying still.

Quality—At first dull and weak, but now it is intense and sharp.

Radiation—The pain started here (pointing to right upper quadrant) and now my shoulder aches.

Severity—On a scale of 1 to 10, it's an 8.

Time/Duration—It started right after dinner and has only gotten worse.

Vital Signs:

Respirations—32 and very shallow

Pulse—Radial pulse bounding at 112 bpm

Blood Pressure—118/76

Temperature—98.2°F (36.8°C)

Pulse Oximetry—96%

Blood Glucose Level—118 mg/dl

Focused Physical Exam (Focused Medical Assessment): Patient remains responsive but unwilling to move extremities because of the increase in abdominal pain.

Differential/Field Diagnosis: Possible gallstones/cholecystitis

Management:
1) High-flow oxygen if tolerated
2) IV access—rehydrate if needed
3) Monitor
4) Transport to appropriate facility

Detailed Physical Exam: En route to appropriate facility as time permits

Ongoing Assessment: There is no change in patient's condition during transport. Maintain position of comfort.

Critical Actions:
1) Keeping patient as still as possible

Teaching Points

1) There are numerous causes and etiologies of chest pain. Assist the participant in classifying chest pain to body system and causes (e.g., cardiac vs. respiratory, trauma vs. medical) for rule outs.

2) Always follow an organized approach to rule out possible causes.

3) Compare and contrast clinical findings of gallstones/cholecystitis to other presentations.

4) Don't let scene clues lead you to a diagnosis preemptively.

5) Discuss visceral versus parietal pain and the progression this patient experienced.

Evaluation

1) *Excellent:* The participant's evaluation of the patient followed set format: initial assessment, focused history (SAMPLE, OPQRST) in an efficient manner. The participant displayed a thorough knowledge of the patient's condition, performed the exam and management in an organized manner, and demonstrated an excellent overall performance.

2) *Good:* The participant's evaluation of the patient followed set format: initial assessment, focused history (SAMPLE, OPQRST) in an acceptable manner with only minor deviation. The participant displayed an above-average knowledge of the patient's condition, performed the exam and management of the patient's condition, and demonstrated an above-average performance.

3) *Fair:* The participant's evaluation of the patient deviated from the set format without causing any further injury to the patient. The participant displayed an average or basic knowledge of the patient's condition and performed an adequate exam and management of the patient's condition.

4) *Inadequate:* The participant's evaluation of the patient deviated significantly from the set format, or the participant's actions endangered the patient's life or significantly exacerbated the condition.

► ACUTE ABDOMINAL PAIN/GI BLEEDING: CASE 4

Requirements: One instructor and one patient for every five participants

Prerequisites: Read Chapter 8, "Acute Abdominal Pain"; Chapter 9, "Gastrointestinal Bleeding"; and Chapter 12, "Headache, Nausea, and Vomiting."

Equipment: One table and chair for the patient to use; jump kit with oxygen supplies (NC, NRM, aerosol mask, PPV device, intubation equipment), stethoscope, BP cuff, cardiac monitor, pulse oximeter, and medication kit with associated medications

Instructor: Your role is vital as your must act as the coordinator of the station and also interact in the scenario. Before the participant arrives at the station, please review the scenario with your patient. Spray the patient's arms with a fine mist of cool water to simulate cool and clammy skin. You will act as the patient's parent who is very concerned. The participant will try to convince you to leave the room so she can get a better history. If she is polite and tactful, you will voluntarily go the other room, but if not, you will become very distraught and will not leave the side of your child. Please read the scenario to become familiar with the necessary responses. Do not "coach" the participant along during the testing station; rather, allow him to conduct the exam without interruption or help.

Patient: One female patient. As the patient, you will be required to play the role of a 16-year-old female complaining of acute abdominal pain. You will be awake and alert and semi-cooperative. You will be reluctant to discuss the possibility of pregnancy unless your parent is removed from the room. Please read the scenario to familiarize yourself with the information. You will have a fine mist of water sprayed on you to simulate cool and diaphoretic skin.

Instructions

Hi, my name is _____ , and I will be the examiner for this station. This is a hands-on patient assessment station. You will be given information concerning a patient experiencing a medical crisis. You will have all the necessary equipment you need to manage the patient in this station. Please look over the equipment before we go any further. You will be provided with pertinent information only when you ask the appropriate question. For any hands-on procedure, such as auscultation of a blood pressure or breath sounds or taking a pulse, select the appropriate equipment needed (if any) and use the equipment in the manner that it would be used on a patient. I will then give you the relevant clinical data. For example, you must select, place, and begin inflation of the BP cuff before the blood pressure is given to you. I will not answer questions in place of the patient. Therefore, it is imperative that you interact with your patient. Please verbalize to me any signs or symptoms that you find so that I will know you are cognizant of the patient and the patient's clinical appearance.

Scenario

Advise the participant that he is responding to a call of a 16-year-old female with abdominal pain who lives in an affluent part of town. If the participant is a nurse or in-hospital provider, the scenario can be modified to the medical environment—such as a new patient with abdominal pain is in Medical Room 5. The participant should use the assessment taught in this course.

Initial Impression: 16-year-old female lying on the bathroom floor on her side

Scene Size-up/General Impression: The scene is safe for entry and exit. No injury is apparent on brief visual exam.

Initial Assessment:

Mental Status—A&O × 3, answering questions

Airway—Clear and patent at this time

Breathing—Respirations 26

Circulation—Radial pulse at 98 bpm

Disability—Moves all four extremities, but reluctantly

Status after Initial Assessment: Serious, potentially unstable

Initial Management Priorities: Oxygen at 15 lpm via NRM, cardiac monitor, IV access

Focused History (SAMPLE):

Signs and Symptoms—Pale, cool and diaphoretic skin; lying on her side in distress

Allergies—Codeine

Medications—Xanax

Past Medical History—Anxiety disorder. If the parent is removed and the patient is asked about pregnancy, she states that she might be.

Last Oral Intake—The patient states that she hasn't consumed anything besides a couple of diet pops over the past 2 days.

Events Preceding—The patient tells you that for the past few days, she has felt worn out, had a loss of appetite, and had a crampy feeling in her lower back. She states that she woke this morning and felt sick to her stomach. She had a couple bouts of nausea and vomiting, and then her lower belly really began to hurt.

OPQRST:

Onset—The pain came on very suddenly.

Palliation/Provocation—It hurts much more when I move.

Quality—The pain was crampy for the past couple of days, but now it is very sharp.

Radiation—I hurt all over, especially in my left shoulder.

Severity—It's really bad now; on a scale of 1 to 10, it's an 8.

Time/Duration—I called for my mom/dad when the pain got worse (20 minutes ago).

Vital Signs:

  Respirations—26 rapid and deep

  Pulse—Radial pulse weak at 98 bpm

  Blood Pressure—86/palp

  Temperature—98.4°F (37°C)

  Pulse Oximetry—94%

  Blood Glucose Level—98 mg/dl

Focused Physical Exam (Focused Medical Assessment): LLQ abdominal pain and guarding

Differential/Field Diagnosis: Abdominal pain; possible ruptured ectopic pregnancy

Management:

  1) High-flow oxygen at 15 lpm via NRM

  2) IV access—fluid bolus to maintain a systolic BP of 70–100 mmHg

  3) Cardiac monitor

  5) Rapid transport to appropriate facility

Detailed Physical Exam: En route to appropriate facility as time permits

Ongoing Assessment: There is no change in patient's condition during transport.

Critical Actions:

  1) Separate parent and child to obtain a thorough history.

  2) Maximize oxygenation with high-flow oxygen.

  3) Place patient in a position of comfort.

Teaching Points

  1) There are numerous causes and etiologies of chest pain. Assist the participant in classifying chest pain to body system and causes (e.g., cardiac vs. respiratory, trauma vs. medical) for rule outs.

  2) Always follow an organized approach to rule out possible causes.

  3) Any female of child bearing age with abdominal pain should be considered to have an ectopic pregnancy until it is ruled out.

  4) Provide rapid transport for surgical emergencies.

Evaluation

  1) *Excellent:* The participant's evaluation of the patient followed set format: initial assessment, focused history (SAMPLE, OPQRST) in an efficient manner. The participant displayed a thorough knowledge of the patient's condition, performed the exam and management in an organized manner, and demonstrated an excellent overall performance.

2) *Good:* The participant's evaluation of the patient followed set format: initial assessment, focused history (SAMPLE, OPQRST) in an acceptable manner with only minor deviation. The participant displayed an above-average knowledge of the patient's condition, performed the exam and management of the patient's condition, and demonstrated an above-average performance.

3) *Fair:* The participant's evaluation of the patient deviated from the set format without causing any further injury to the patient. The participant displayed an average or basic knowledge of the patient's condition and performed an adequate exam and management of the patient's condition.

4) *Inadequate:* The participant's evaluation of the patient deviated significantly from the set format, or the participant's actions endangered the patient's life or significantly exacerbated the condition.

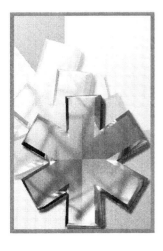

IV. AMLS
INSTRUCTOR COURSE

⊞ ADMINISTRATION

The purpose of the AMLS Instructor Course is to provide the AMLS Instructor/ Coordinator candidate with the knowledge, skills, and support materials necessary to conduct and/or participate as faculty in an approved AMLS course.

Setting/Time

The course is ideally conducted at the conclusion of an AMLS Provider Course. The Instructor Course may be taken before or after a Provider Course, depending on the audience. The course is designed to be a case-based, interactive lecture format. The course is approved for 4 hours of continuing education by the Continuing Education Coordinating Board of Emergency Medical Services (CECBEMS) and the National Association of Emergency Medical Technicians (NAEMT) Education Accreditation Committee.

Standardization

It is essential to disseminate the course philosophy and content consistent with the standards established by the NAEMT, the AMLS Executive Council, and the CECBEMS. No deviations in content are recommended. Any removal or addition of slides, equipment, materials, or structure of the Instructor Course requires approval in advance and in writing to the NAEMT Executive Council and the AMLS Executive Council. Approval should not be assumed. Approval, if granted, will be submitted in writing to the requesting individual.

Materials

Each Instructor/Coordinator candidate is required to have a copy of the *AMLS Coordinator and Instructor Guide,* 2nd Ed.

Surcharge/Costs

The surcharge for the Instructor Course is payable to NAEMT in the amount of $10/participant. The host organization is responsible for all course fees. Participant fees are determined at the discretion of the host organization.

Post-course Materials

The following post-course materials should be sent to NAEMT headquarters within 30 days of completion of the course:

- ▶ Participant roster
- ▶ Course evaluations
- ▶ Appropriate surcharge for number of participants
- ▶ Resume/curriculum vitae for each participant as an instructor
- ▶ Information that indicates each participant successfully completed the Instructor/Coordinator program.

Instructor Course Faculty

Each course will be conducted with at least one AMLS national or Affiliate Faculty. The total number of the faculty will be at the discretion of the national or Affiliate Faculty.

Instructor/Coordinator Candidates

Each Instructor/Coordinator candidate

- ▶ Will have completed an AMLS Provider Course within the last year.
- ▶ Must present a resume and/or curriculum vitae and copies of their Provider Course completion card.
- ▶ Must have a minimum of one year experience in teaching advanced levels of healthcare providers. Prehospital Trauma Life Support (PHTLS) or Pediatric Prehospital Care (PPC) instructor experience is recommended.

Upon completion of the Instructor/Coordinator Course, the participant will be considered an Instructor candidate. Each Instructor candidate will receive an Instructor Course completion certificate. Each candidate will be monitored by recognized AMLS Affiliate Faculty within one year of the Instructor/Coordinator course. The Affiliate Faculty that monitors the Instructor candidate will submit the satisfactory instructor monitor form with the post-course paperwork for the Associate Provider course. The Affiliate Faculty will issue an AMLS instructor card.

Objectives

At the completion of the Instructor/Coordinator Course, the participant will be able to:

1) Identify the components of the AMLS organizational structure.

2) Identify the AMLS Executive Council.

3) Access the NAEMT headquarters by phone, fax, or E-mail.

4) Complete the pre- and post-course materials for course coordination.

5) Explain the rationale for the questions on the AMLS pretest and post-test written evaluation.

6) Discuss the AMLS conceptual approach to medical emergencies by moving the healthcare provider from an initial assessment to a diagnostic model by enhancing critical thinking skills.

7) Understand how educational guidance to the healthcare provider can provide a better link to differential diagnoses by avoiding faulty conclusions that are sometimes reached even though the provider is experienced.

8) Discuss the AMLS course philosophy, goals, objectives, format, and required curriculum; AV materials coordination; use of victims/patients; and how to enhance case-scenario practice in group settings.

9) Discuss the levels of achievement in health care—from the novice to the expert level—and how healthcare providers can teach peers to help each other by using the critical thinking process.

Instructor/Coordinator Course Agenda

0845   Registration

0900   Welcome/Introduction

       AMLS Author Considerations and the AMLS Textbook

       Goals and Objectives of AMLS

1000   Break

1010   Course Philosophy

       The Links: Moving the Practitioner From Assessment to Diagnostic Model

       Inductive Thinking—From Novice to Expert—Critical Thinking Skills

1100   Break

1110   How to Coordinate the AMLS Course (Use of the AMLS Coordinator and Instructor Guide)

       How to Coordinate and Use Audio Visual Aids

       How to Conduct and Enhance Case Studies Through Group Practice Scenarios

       The Role of the Instructor/Coordinator and Faculty Members

1200   Evaluation and Adjourn

▦ AMLS INSTRUCTOR COURSE SLIDE NOTES

SLIDE NO.   **SLIDE TITLE/NOTES**

Slide I-1   **AMLS Instructor Workshop**
- ▶ Faculty member should review the prerequisites for the AMLS instructor program at this time:
  - — Healthcare instructor program that includes the principles of adult education. Example: ACLS Instructor, PALS Instructor, PHTLS Instructor, EMS Instructor, etc.
  - — Score at least 84% on the final written AMLS Provider exam
  - — Has years of experience in the emergency healthcare setting (resume to Coordinator)
  - — Has working knowledge of anatomy, physiology, and pathophysiology

Slide I-2   **Instructor Course Objectives**

Slide I-3   **Objectives (continued)**

Slide I-4   **The Authors of the AMLS Text**
- ▶ Each of the authors possesses a wealth of knowledge and experience in emergency medicine and healthcare education.
- ▶ The AMLS text includes the E-mail address of each author.

Slide I-5   **The Assumptions Made . . .**
- ▶ The AMLS text and the course were designed with the assumption that even though experience is the best teacher, some links between a standard medical patient assessment and what the provider decides is a plan of care (mostly based on protocols) can be incorrect.
- ▶ For instance: When confronted with a patient with a complaint of dyspnea who is wheezing, what does the novice provider assess and conclude? What does the experienced provider do?

Slide I-6   **The AMLS Text**
- ▶ The AMLS text is based on the written assumptions that we need a better approach to our assessment, more tools at our disposal to make an initial impression, and the knowledge that our initial impression must include a list of differential diagnoses with a fluid approach to ruling them in or out as we manage the patient.
- ▶ This is the kind of approach that a seasoned veteran would use!

Slide I-7   **The AMLS Text (continued)**
- ▶ All healthcare professionals need to be taught the process of forming an initial impression and listing differential diagnoses.
- ▶ The participants in this program need a strong knowledge base in anatomy, physiology, and pathophysiology, as well as a scenario-based format to reinforce the inductive process needed for the diagnosis-based style of emergency patient care.

▶ Experienced emergency care providers will also appreciate this professional style of patient assessment and management.

Slide I-8   **Goals of the AMLS Text**

▶ The chapters in the AMLS text review the basics of adult medical emergency assessment and management.

▶ The patient assessment chapter of the text is a key element in the process of moving from the outmoded assessment-based model to the diagnosis-based method of patient management.

▶ Each chapter presents an integrated, practical approach in medical diagnoses. Instruction progresses from the complaint-based, assessment-based initial assessment to the field-diagnosis and management format.

▶ Chapter 1 guides participants through the concepts. Each chapter is focused on a common medical complaint and is presented in an integrated, practical approach.

▶ Appendices provide reference information.

Slide I-9   **AMLS Course Philosophy**

Slide I-10   **AMLS Course Philosophy**

▶ Participant prerequisites should include education in anatomy, physiology, and pathophysiology with experience in an emergency medicine setting.

▶ The program is geared to the advanced-level provider.

Slide I-11   **AMLS Course Philosophy (continued)**

▶ Scenarios teach the diagnosis-based method, then allow the participant to apply the method as he/she is guided through successes and failures. Critical thinking skills are key!

Slide I-12   **Field Thinking Process**

▶ How do emergency medicine/EMS providers think when confronted with an emergency patient?
  — They gather some information.
  — They use their base knowledge in anatomy, physiology, and pathophysiology.
  — Their personal attitude toward their profession is included within their base knowledge: complacency, paranoia, etc.
  — Experience level and knowledge of what their Medical Director wants is taken into account.
  — They then apply whatever protocol seems appropriate.
    ▪ If they are competent, they reassess the patient to make sure that the protocol worked.
    ▪ They learn from their mistakes (if guided appropriately).
    ▪ They learn more as they reflect on formal and informal processes.

	SLIDE NO.	SLIDE TITLE/NOTES
	Slide I-13	**Field Thinking Process**

Field Thinking Process
- If the providers are competent, they realize that the protocol chosen was not right, try a different approach, and with guidance gain more experience.
- Formal process of run critique (if done appropriately) will also provide guided education.
- Ultimately, this process leads to the inductive method of education through experience.

Slide I-14   **Novice to Expert**
- Review the different levels of provider in the emergency healthcare setting . . . from novice to expert.
- Reinforce this professional knowledge. Professionals should mentor the novice and guide them to learn from experience.

Slide I-15   **The Novice**
- Entry-level
- Has extensive book knowledge, but needs hands-on experience
- Someone who has a good education can enter the work force at the advanced beginner stage. However, if the graduate paramedic was placed in an ICU in the hospital—he or she would be a novice.

Slide I-16   **The Advanced Beginner**
- Has enough experience to be able to piece some blocks of information together but still has difficulty distinguishing between relevant and irrelevant information. (Is still a list follower.)
- This is usually the level one finds in the graduate paramedic, especially if she/he comes from an education program in which numerous case scenarios are managed.

Slide I-17   **The Competent Level**
- Can see the uniqueness of a situation—sees that it is not quite right, but still depends on the "rules" for dealing with a specific disease process and follows the set pattern.
  — Is competent, but can't think outside the box. Is able to distinguish between relevant and irrelevant information during the healthcare process.

Slide I-18   **The Proficient Level**
- Able to gather blocks of information, weed out the irrelevant and the unique, and recall experiences from past events. Begins to see special situations earlier and with more experienced eyes.
- Sees the overall picture; has intuition.

Slide I-19   **The Expert Level**
- Able to recognize the patient in congestive heart failure by taking one look at the patient and without asking questions.
- Able to determine that a patient in the nursing home who has a sudden onset of shortness of breath accompanied by a cough as possibly having aspiration pneumonia and asks the right questions to rule it in.

▶ Often has correct "hunches" or gut feelings. This person would be a great mentor, as long as he/she can break down critical thinking skills for the learner.

▶ Uses analytic tools when a situation does not turn out as planned or when faced with a new situation.

NOTE: You may have six, three-person groups in your AMLS class comprised of 10 novices (students in a paramedic class) and 8 experienced EMS providers who are at proficient and expert levels. How would you combine the groups?

Slide I-20   **Revisiting the Field Thinking Process**
▶ Combining the levels of experience with the field thinking process revisits how a protocol is chosen *or* how a field impression is formed.

Slide I-21   **Field Thinking Process (continued)**
▶ Segue to next slide at the end of this discussion . . .we will now discuss how to coordinate an AMLS course.

Slide I-22   **Course Coordination**

Slide I-23   **NAEMT**
▶ The National Association of EMTs sets the rules and administers the AMLS course, along with PHTLS and PPC.
▶ The National Association of EMS Physicians endorses this course for medical content and quality assurance.

Slide I-24   **The Coordinator and Instructor Guide**
▶ Slides and Instructor Notes within this Guide along with the rules of course coordination:
— Set of slides purchased from Brady Publishing
— The AMLS Provider/Refresher Courses may be used outside the AMLS course.
— New set of case-based lecture slide presentations have been revised and are available with the *Coordinator and Instructor Guide,* 2nd ed.
— These new slides are from NAEMT for AMLS instructors.

Slide I-25   **Coordination of the Provider Course**
▶ This course cannot be conducted without providing the AMLS text to each participant and emphasizing the importance of reading it prior to the course. The cover letter, AMLS text, and pretest should be sent to the preregistered participants at least one month in advance.
▶ This course is written for the advanced level EMS provider but can easily be used for flight nurses and emergency medicine nurses. For example, scenarios allude to the ED triage desk and the instructor must follow that format throughout the case for that team or team leader.

Slide I-26   **The AMLS Refresher Course**
▶ The new Refresher Course agenda is included in Part V of this Guide.

▸ The agenda includes a review of initial impression and differential diagnoses within the patient assessment presentation and medical emergency case studies managed with moulaged victims.

Slide I-27 **AMLS Refresher Course**

▸ The 4-hour AMLS Refresher Course is described as either an independent course or built within the 2nd day of the Provider Course.
— For those at the end of the 3-year certification period (no grace)

▸ Includes a 2-hour review of the 5 main topics of AMLS: Hypoperfusion, Dyspnea, Chest Pain, Altered Mental Status, and Abdominal Pain/GI Bleeding with emphasis on the AMLS concept of medical patient assessment (i.e., use of initial impressions and differential diagnoses)
— There is one case study per topic, with participant discussion integral to the review session.
— The instructor then reviews the pretest with the participants.
— The participants then are organized into groups for exam rotations—Case 4 of each of the four main topics: Dyspnea, Chest Pain (which includes shock), Altered Mental Status, Abdominal Pain/GI Bleeding; along with the written exam.
— Successful completion allows another 3 years of AMLS certification

Slide I-28 **AMLS Affiliate Faculty**

▸ Each international country and U.S. state will have at least one Affiliate Faculty, depending on geographic concerns and course activity.

▸ The role of the Affiliate Faculty includes quality assurance and course administration for NAEMT.

Slide I-29 **Affiliate Faculty Qualifications**

▸ A listing of the Affiliate Faculty qualifications
— Each applicant for Affiliate Faculty will be reviewed by the NAEMT AMLS Executive Council.
— Experience in teaching, course administration, and quality assurance will be considered along with recommendations from National Committee members.

Slide I-30 **Course Coordinator for AMLS**

▸ The key to the success of an AMLS course is the local coordinator. This *AMLS Coordinator and Instructor Guide* provides guidance for the paperwork and rules of the course, but the coordinator needs to organize, advertise, and administer the course's daily operations. Upon course completion, the coordinator completes and sends the final course paperwork to the NAEMT office.

▸ We recommend that new instructors do not attempt to become course coordinators in their first AMLS course. Please ask for assistance from local course coordinators and Affiliate Faculty members.

Slide I-31 **Coordinator Qualifications**

Slide I-32 **Job Description of the AMLS Course Coordinator**

Slide I-33 **AMLS Instructor**
▸ Review the prerequisites for AMLS instructor
— The Affiliate Faculty who monitors the new AMLS Instructor will send a packet of information to the NAEMT office upon satisfaction of the requirements.
— This packet includes the new instructor's resume, a letter of recommendation from the AMLS Provider course coordinator/director, a letter of recommendation from the instructor's Medical Director, and the 2-sided AMLS Instructor Monitor form completed by the Affiliate Faculty.
— The AMLS instructor should teach at least one course per year.

Slide I-34 **Instructor Qualifications**
▸ Review of the prerequisites for the AMLS instructor

Slide I-35 **Duties of the AMLS Instructor**
▸ The AMLS instructor must follow the rules of the NAEMT and the course authors who encourage inductive methods in case-based teaching and the development of critical thinking skills.
▸ During a course, instructors operate as a team and discuss how well the participants (as a whole and individually) are doing with the concepts and philosophy of the program.
▸ Experienced instructors should eventually be able to present several of the lectures within this program.

Slide I-36 **Course Medical Director**
▸ In charge of the medical content presented during the program, so has an integral duty in choosing who should present the information (i.e., faculty).
▸ Should always be available for any questions that may arise about medical content or with administrative rules (along with the Affiliate Faculty).

Slide I-37 **Qualifications of Medical Director**
▸ Must be a licensed physician in the geographic region of the course with an active interest in emergency medicine and with special knowledge in EMS. This is important because he/she is the resource person (along with Affiliate Faculty) for the course while adhering to NAEMT/AMLS course guidelines and standards.

Slide I-38   **Participant Prerequisites**
▶ Segue into participant prerequisites for the program.

Slide I-39   **Participant Prerequisites**
▶ This course is written for the advanced level of EMS or emergency medicine healthcare provider which presumes experience and knowledge in anatomy, physiology, and pathophysiology.
▶ Many training programs use this course design, adapt the agenda, and include it toward the end of their National Standard Paramedic curriculum. It is used to summarize the medical emergencies sections and provides a forum for critical thinking skills labs in a case-scenario format.
▶ Basic level participants can "certify" in this course but need to take the basic level final written exam.

Slide I-40   **Participant to Instructor Ratio**
▶ There should be one instructor for every 5 participants for each case scenario. There should be one instructor for every 2–3 participants for the final exam rotations.

Slide I-41   **Course Schedule**
▶ Some minor adaptations of the agenda can be done once the initial assessment and airway lectures are completed, but the lecture must precede any case study topics in the group rotations.
▶ The Affiliate Faculty and Medical Director should be made aware of any changes in the agenda.

Slide I-42   **Course Paperwork and Coordination**
▶ See Part VII in this Guide for the course application and budget forms.
  — These two forms, plus a proposed agenda with faculty assignments should be sent to the NAEMT office (and Affiliate Faculty) 60 days prior to the course.
  — The office will send out a course packet which includes pretest, post-test, and answer keys/reference sheets, certificates, and cards prior to the course.
  — There will be some handouts for participants that may be used for math in drug calculations. There is a reference handout for SAMPLE and OPQRST history gathering in the initial assessment included in the packet.
▶ The office will also send an invoice with the National Course Number assigned. The region's Affiliate Faculty may assign the State Course Number.
▶ Each participant should complete the information requested on the application found at the back of this Guide. Participants can preregister or register on the first day of class.
▶ The NAEMT surcharge fee is $15 per participant for the Provider Course, $10 per participant for the Refresher Course, and $10 per participant for the Instructor Course. Surcharge fees should be sent to NAEMT with course paperwork within 1 week following the course.

Slide I-43   **Continuing Education for AMLS**
- ▶ If no local EMS continuing education underwriter is available to the course coordinator, contact the CECBEMS. NAEMT has picked up the cost of this resource.
- ▶ Most states approve this program for continuing education for nurses as well.
- ▶ The coordinator should investigate whether this program could be assigned college credit through the college of his or her choice.

Slide I-44   **Participant Packet**
- ▶ Review of the participant packet (discussed earlier, along with the importance of reading the AMLS textbook)

Slide I-45   **Case Scenarios**
- ▶ Segue to a new discussion on how to conduct the group case scenarios.

Slide I-46   **Group Activity**
- ▶ A review of how the practice and testing scenarios are chosen for each topic
- ▶ Case 4 of each topic is used to test participants in the Refresher Course.

Slide I-47   **Group Activity**
- ▶ Instructors should read over each case assigned to them, organize the equipment, and prepare (moulage) the patient.
- ▶ Directions to the participants should include that a hands-on medical assessment and history gathering will be expected, using AMLS principles. Each participant should take turns playing the role of team member and team leader as they practice—and test.

Slide I-48   **Group Activity**
- ▶ Have teams look over their equipment and go over last-minute instructions.
  - — The patient should assume the role described in the scenario and the instructor should read the scenario information.
  - — The first scenario of the course should be conducted slowly and should allow for some interruptions. The remaining scenarios should be conducted as is.

Slide I-49   **The Initial Scenario Conducted for a Group**
- ▶ The first round of scenarios conducted for the assigned groups should be done in order to reinforce the principles of forming an initial impression with a list of differentials that can be ruled in and out.
- ▶ The instructor may let the group get started with its initial assessment—stop, and . . .

Ask: *Is this patient stable or unstable?*

Ask: *Should you go ahead and obtain a history or did your initial assessment indicate resuscitation is needed immediately?*
What's next?

▶ After some assessment is completed . . .

Ask: *What is your field impression at this point?*
— Ask each team member.
▶ Compile the list of differentials or ask the group what its list should include.

Ask: *What should you do with this information?*
What's next?
▶ Continue this format as participants compile information that leads toward a successful field impression with accompanying appropriate management.
▶ This is the LAST time you will conduct this type of group scenarios. From this point on, the groups will perform as if they were on a real call—no input will be given by the instructor other than answers to questions not answered through conversation with the prepared patient.

Slide I-50   Initial Group Activity (continued)
▶ Initial scenario, as described earlier. The field thinking process enforces critical thinking skills throughout the first round of scenarios.

Slide I-51   Initial Group Activity (continued)
▶ As described before, only the initial group rounds perform the cases step by step with instructor assistance.

Slide I-52   Group Activity
▶ The group may use their handouts (provided by NAEMT) as a reminder of the OPQRST and SAMPLE questions that should be asked.
▶ The instructor should provide positive reinforcement at the end of each case presentation and remind participants of the importance of good history-taking in order to form a correct field impression and effective management plan.

NOTE: If the team leader (especially a proficient or expert level provider) completed the scenario with a high level of success—quickly formed the correct field impression—have the leader review HOW he/she came to this correct impression. Guided review of this process is excellent for the novices or beginners in the group as well as the higher functioning providers.

Slide I-53   Common Mistakes in Group Activity
▶ Let the groups make these mistakes but review them upon summary.
▶ If a group leader incorrectly guides the participants through an incorrect field impression or differential diagnosis, the instructor should review the team's dynamics and AMLS assessment format.

Slide I-54   **Group Activity—Management**
▶ Critique upon completion of each scenario. Lead discussions with the group—do not lecture.
▶ Each diagnosis should be reviewed using appropriate anatomy and pathophysiology terminology.
▶ Instructors: Avoid tunnel vision. There is more than one way to do most things. Keep reinforcing the principles of AMLS—don't get bogged down on management.

Slide I-55   **Final Evaluation**
▶ Final Written Exam: Passing score of 80%
▶ May retest after remediation from the instructor.

Slide I-56   **Final Evaluation (continued)**
▶ Have the groups rotate through the final case scenarios with each participant taking turns being team member and team leader.
▶ The instructor at each station must document each team's performance on the form provided.
▶ Two scenarios have been chosen for testing. Use the second one if the group needs to demonstrate meeting the objectives with another case. Remediate before retesting.

Slide I-57   **Questions?**
Any questions?

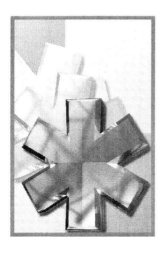

V. AMLS REFRESHER COURSE

⊞ ADMINISTRATION

The purpose of the AMLS Refresher Course is to review and enhance the content of the AMLS Provider Course and to reaffirm its knowledge and key skill components.

Term of AMLS Recognition

The term of AMLS certificate/card recognition is three years. It is recommended that a refresher class be taken no later than three years from the original Provider Course or three years from the last Refresher Course.

Certificates of completion and wallet cards are issued by the Course Coordinator and/or Affiliate Faculty upon successful completion of the Refresher Course.

If an individual is unable to take a Refresher Course, Coordinators and Affiliate Faculty can admit an individual into a scheduled Refresher Course for up to six months past his/her expiration date if the participant's Medical Director requests in writing that the individual maintain an AMLS provider status. This will not change or alter the individual's expiration date; it will only reflect an extended period within which an individual will be allowed into a Refresher Course. Participants who are seeking to reinstate their term of recognition after their expiration date are required to attend a full Provider Course.

Prerequisite Requirement for Participants

Each participant in the AMLS Refresher Course must have successfully completed an AMLS Provider Course within the last three years. Each participant must have maintained his/her certification/licensure as an advanced skilled EMT-Basic, advanced healthcare provider, paramedic, nurse, physician assistant, or physician.

Setting/Time

The course is ideally conducted as a stand alone four-hour course. The course is approved for 4 hours of continuing education credit through CECBEMS. The Refresher Course can be taught in conjunction with the second day of the Provider Course. This compatibility will allow for participants from the provider and refresher courses to participate in the evaluation stations simultaneously. Each evaluation station should have one instructor and one individual to serve as the patient.

Materials

Each participant should have a copy of the current edition of the *Advanced Medical Life Support* textbook and pre-course materials included in the Provider Course. Pre-course materials should be sent to the participants a minimum of 30 days prior to the course date. In addition, evaluation station equipment should be available for the following stations: Chest Pain Case 4, Dyspnea Case 4, Altered Mental Status Case 4, and Abdominal Pain/GI Bleeding Case 4. Hypoperfusion information is also evaluated in Chest Pain Case 4.

Standardization

It is essential to disseminate the course philosophy and content consistent with the standards established by the NAEMT, the AMLS Executive Council, and the CECBEMS. No deviations in content are recommended. Any removal or addition of slides, equipment, materials, or structure of the Refresher Course requires approval in advance and in writing to the NAEMT Executive Council and the AMLS Executive Council. Approval should not be assumed. Approval, if granted, will be submitted in writing to the requesting individual.

Course Application

The AMLS Refresher Course application process will follow the same procedure as a provider course.

Surcharge/Costs

The surcharge for the Refresher Course is payable to NAEMT in the amount of $10/participant and should be included with post-course materials. The host organization is responsible for all course fees.

Participant fees are determined at the discretion of the host organization.

Post-course Materials

The following post-course materials should be sent to the NAEMT headquarters within 30 days of completion of the course.

▶ Participant roster

▶ Course evaluation

▶ Evidence that each participant met the competency requirements for all the evaluation stations

▶ Appropriate surcharge for each participant

Refresher Course Faculty

Recognized AMLS Instructors and Affiliate Faculty are eligible to instruct the Refresher Course.

Objectives

At the completion of the AMLS Refresher Course the participant will be able to:

1) Review the key concepts of the AMLS Provider Course.

2) Expand the participant's knowledge and understanding of the key concepts learned in the AMLS Provider Course as it is revised based on new research and changes in medicine related to the adult medical patient.

3) Reaffirm that the participant has the content knowledge and ability to perform the key skills identified in the AMLS case scenarios with competency.

4) Maintain their AMLS Provider recognition for an additional three-year term.

AMLS Refresher Course Agenda

(Incorporated with second day of Provider Course using Schedule A):

0830   Registration

0900   Welcome/Introduction

0915   AMLS Refresher Review Presentation—Part I

1020   Break

1035   AMLS Refresher Review Presentation—Part II

1135   Review of Pretest

1200   Lunch

1245   Group Evaluation Rotations in Dyspnea, Chest Pain, Altered Mental Status, and Abdominal Pain/GI Bleeding. (Case 4 will be used for all evaluation stations. Chest Pain Case 4 encompasses hypoperfusion. Case 3 can be used for retesting situations after remediation.)

The Written Exam is also taken at an evaluation station.

1545   Course Evaluation/ Cards Awarded

(Incorporated with second day of Provider Course using Schedule B):

0815   Registration

0845   Welcome/Introduction

0900   AMLS Refresher Review Presentation—Part I

1000   Break

1015   AMLS Refresher Review Presentation—Part II

1115   Review of Pretest

1200   Lunch

1245   Group Evaluation Rotations in Dyspnea, Chest Pain, Altered Mental Status, and Abdominal Pain/GI Bleeding. (Case 4 will be used for all evaluation stations. Chest Pain Case 4 encompasses hypoperfusion. Case 3 can be used for retesting situations after remediation.)

The Written Exam is also an evaluation station.

1545   Course Evaluation/Cards Awarded

Stand Alone Course

0730   Registration

0800   Welcome/Introduction

0810   AMLS Refresher Review Presentation—Part I

0900   Break

0910   AMLS Refresher Review Presentation—Part II

1010   Break

1020   Review of Pretest

1030   Group Evaluation Rotations in Dyspnea, Chest Pain, Altered Mental Status, and Abdominal Pain/GI Bleed. (Case 4 will be used for all evaluation stations. Chest Pain Case 4 encompasses hypoperfusion. Case 3 can be used for retesting situations after remediation.)

1130   Written Exam

1215   Course Evaluation/Cards Awarded

SLIDE NO.   **SLIDE TITLE/NOTES**

Slide R-1   **NAEMT**

Sponsored by the National Association of EMTs, this is a four-hour program designed for those participants who completed the Advanced Medical Life Support (AMLS) Provider Course three years ago.

Slide R-2   **AMLS Refresher Review**

The first two hours of this program is designed to review the medical patient assessment in two parts via case studies. We will then review the pretest, the testing of scenarios, and the written exam.

Slide R-3   **Objectives**

Paraphrase the objectives of this two-part initial session for the AMLS Refresher Course.

Slide R-4   **Components of Assessment**

▶ The components of the medical patient assessment are staged into five essential steps with many secondary components within the steps.

▶ Decide whether this is a medical or a trauma call based on both dispatch information and as part of scene size-up. With confusing situations, the ability to determine whether the case is medical or trauma may have to wait until the focused history and physical exam.

▶ Identify and manage immediate life threats in the initial assessment. This, along with the scene size-up, helps you determine whether this patient is stable or unstable and whether you should proceed to aggressive resuscitation or have time to perform a focused history and physical exam.

▶ Gather a patient history and perform a physical exam that is centered around the patient's chief complaint, even if unconsciousness is that complaint.

▶ Perform a detailed physical exam with vital signs.

▶ Provide continued and advanced medical care based on your differential impressions and continuously monitor the patient's condition with assessment of whether your treatment was effective. Communicate and document this information.

Slide R-5   **Scene Size-up**

▶ Based on dispatch information, begin to develop a mental list of possibilities as to what's wrong with a patient. This continues as you approach and enter the scene. Scene size-up is the initial evaluation of the scene and the patient within it.

— What body substance precautions should I take?

— What hazards (or potential hazards) may be present?

▪ Ensure safety of self, partner, patient, and bystanders

— What other resources do I need to call for on this scene?

▪ Is this a medical or trauma patient?

▶ The scene size-up should be continuously re-evaluated.

	SLIDE NO.	SLIDE TITLE/NOTES

Slide R-6 **Stable/Unstable**

▶ Is this patient physiologically stable or unstable? (Many times categorized by the seasoned EMS provider subconsciously: "Sick or not sick?")

▶ Stable means no immediate life threats. Unstable means that the patient is in need of immediate intervention, possibly early transport.

▶ This question is usually answered through assessment of the initial ABCD.

▶ Patient must be continuously reassessed.

▶ Look for the "red flags" of instability during the initial assessment.

Slide R-7 **Instability**

▶ Airway: Any sounds or signs of airway obstruction are key signs of instability.

▶ This would warrant immediate interventions prior to moving on to any other portion of the assessment.

Slide R-8 **Instability**

▶ Breathing: The general rate and work of breathing are assessed for "sick or not sick."

▶ Any accessory muscle use, poor air movement, irregular patterns, or extremes in rate (bradypnea or tachypnea) are all signs that the patient needs immediate interventions.

Slide R-9 **Instability**

▶ Circulation: Key indicators of instability within the circulatory assessment include these criteria.

▶ The assessment must include checking peripheral and central pulses, as well as skin vitals.

Slide R-10 **Instability**

▶ CNS: A sense of low Glasgow Coma score, with emphasis on the AVPU, no spontaneous movement or inability to move extremities to command

Slide R-11 **Initial Assessment**

▶ Recaps what has been done so far in our medical patient assessment.

▶ Prioritization and initial management are completed before we move on to gaining a history and performing a detailed physical assessment.

▶ In some patient situations, immediate transport may also need to be done.

Slide R-12 **History**

▶ The OPQRST format guides the provider in gathering a thorough history of the chief complaint.

▶ It is centered on the complaint of pain or discomfort but can certainly be used for a dyspnea scale in those patients who are chronically or intermittently short of breath.

NOTE: If the patient indicates that his dyspnea is a high number on the scale, the provider should ask what happened the last time the patient's feelings of dyspnea were this severe (e.g., intubation, hospitalization).

Slide R-13   Associated Complaints
▶ Associated complaints are derived through direct questions. For instance, with a chief complaint of chest pain, the provider should ask direct questions as to whether the patient is having difficulty breathing, nausea, weakness, lightheadedness, or palpitations.
▶ If the patient denies these associated complaints, they are communicated and documented as pertinent negatives.

Slide R-14   SAMPLE
▶ Gain information on the patient's past medical history with use of the SAMPLE mnemonic. This helps you remember the pertinent questions.
▶ Make sure to ask about over-the-counter (OTC) medications as well as prescribed medications.
— OTC medications include herbs and supplements.
▶ Obtain surgical and hospitalization history.

Slide R-15   Unresponsive History
▶ When the patient is unable to provide a history due to altered mental status, this becomes the chief complaint. AMS makes it even more imperative to gain clues from the environment. This patient is also considered unstable.

Slide R-16   Focused Physical Exam
▶ Perform a focused physical exam that is specific to the chief complaint.
— Thorough head-to-toe assessment for unconscious patients
▶ DO NOT develop tunnel vision while forming your initial impression.
— EXAMPLE: I'm sure this patient who is having abdominal pain has cholecystitis, so I'm only going to examine the abdomen.

Slide R-17   Ongoing Assessment
▶ A physical assessment is a continuous process. The ongoing assessment is completed after the focused history and physical exam and after initial management techniques.
▶ Re-evaluation is completed at routine intervals, based on the stability of the patient's condition.
▶ A final impression may not be formed until more diagnostic studies are completed in a definitive area of the hospital.
▶ Avoid tunnel vision.

Slide R-18   Initial Impression
▶ The AMLS process of forming an initial impression . . .
— What could be wrong with this patient? (initial impression)
— What else could be wrong? (differential diagnoses)
▶ The process of forming the initial impression is based on the steps of the AMLS patient assessment.

▸ Experience on the part of the provider, an open attitude, and team collaboration are helpful in this process.

▸ Develop a treatment plan and re-evaluate whether the patient is getting better or worse and whether your initial impression needs to be revised.

▸ The process described is from the beginning to end of the call but the process continues into retrospective call review and continuing education within quality improvement activities.

NOTE: Segue into Case Study 1: We're now going to review the process of AMLS assessment, forming an initial impression with discussion of the clues to ruling in or ruling out the differentials of "What is wrong with this patient?".

Slide R-19   **Case Study 1: Unknown Etiology**
NOTE: Teach the participants how these cases will be presented throughout this program. Audience participation is a must. Slides won't be advanced until the entire audience gets involved in answering questions and discussing procedures.

Slide R-20   **Case Study 1: Scene Size-up**
▸ Paraphrase the information on the slide. (DO NOT READ TO THE PARTICIPANTS.)

Ask: *Does this scene appear safe?*
Does this appear to be a medical or a trauma patient?
From the doorway, does this patient appear to be stable or unstable?
— Reinforced answers: This appears to be a safe medical scene so far. There doesn't appear to be a need for additional resources as yet. The patient's work of breathing is a red flag for instability of breathing.

NOTE: DO NOT advance to the next slide until the participants provide potential answers. Provide positive feedback for all responses and guide correct ones.

Slide R-21   **Case Study 1: Initial Assessment**
▸ Look for life threats and intervene if necessary.
▸ Paraphrase this information.

Ask: *What may be wrong with this patient?*
What else could be wrong?
Possibilities?
— Reinforced answers: This patient is considered to be hypoperfused with difficulty breathing.
— The possibilities might include: acute MI, cardiogenic shock, GI bleed, sepsis, pulmonary embolus, etc.

NOTE: DO NOT move to next slide until this slide has been discussed BY THE PARTICIPANTS!
▸ Segue to next slide by introducing the subject of shock or hypoperfusion and the key points in deciding the cause of the shock (differentials).

Slide R-22 **Shock**
▶ Hypoperfusion is inadequate tissue perfusion, localized or systemic. The term shock is synonymous with systemic hypoperfusion, which can lead to death if untreated.
▶ There are a variety of causes but generally results from problems with lungs, heart, blood vessels, blood, or nervous system.

Slide R-23 **Shock Differential**
▶ Differential diagnoses in shock:
— Based on the organ you find involved (e.g., crackles heard in bases of lung fields may indicate cardiogenic shock).
— The differentials are based on pump (heart), pipes (vessels), or volume.

Slide R-24 **Shock Types**
▶ The four categories of shock include:
— Hypovolemic (which includes blood loss from medical etiologies, GI fluid loss)
— Obstructive (that which obstructs blood flow around the heart and lungs)
— Distributive (vessels affected by size or leakage)
— Cardiogenic
▶ We learn the signs and symptoms of shock based on the findings in hemorrhagic shock. Review the signs and symptoms of the different categories of shock, comparing them to hemorrhagic shock signs and symptoms.

Slide R-25 **Shock Signs**
▶ Non-hemorrhagic shock signs vs. hemorrhagic shock table

NOTE: The table slides can be a bit confusing. It is important to highlight key points for participants.

▶ Clues/Differentials:
— Hypovolemic shock, whether from blood loss or volume loss through GI or other causes, exhibits the classic signs of shock with the body's attempt to compensate by conserving water
▪ Creates oliguria, poor tissue hydration, and thirst.
— Note that in the elderly, the thirst mechanism has been altered due to natural aging, which adds to the significance of hypovolemia in that age group.
▪ Skin vitals in dehydration vary from classic signs— sweating may not be as apparent and the skin may tent.

Slide R-26 **Shock—Obstructive Causes**
▶ Obstructive shock is caused by any condition that inhibits preload or afterload of the heart.
▶ Each of these causes of obstructive shock will be discussed individually and the signs and symptoms compared to classic hemorrhagic shock (because that's the way wc remember them).

Shock—Pulmonary Emboli

▶ Pulmonary emboli interferes with preload to the left ventricle.

▶ Clues/Differentials:

— Chest pain does not always occur; however, if it does, it is often pleuritic.

— Patient has a sense of impending doom due to brainstem hypoxia.

— Tachycardia is due to decreased blood flow in the chest and tachypnea is due to hypoxia.

— Lung sounds are usually clear but depend on the "clot shower."

— Syncope and/or cardiac arrest may occur depending on the clot shower distribution.

— Skin vitals range from pallor to cyanosis or grayness, especially around the nose and mouth.

— The emboli triggers an inflammatory response that can create dysrhythmias, especially PVCs and atrial fibrillation.

Shock—Cardiac Tamponade

▶ Cardiac tamponade interferes with both preload and after-load—usually associated with trauma but rarely can occur with medical conditions.

▶ The pathophysiology is restriction of cardiac filling caused by accumulation of fluid in the pericardium.

▶ Can be caused by large pericardial effusions from leukemia and certain other chronic conditions

▶ Clues/Differentials:

— Pulsus paradoxus

— Neck and hand vein distension

— A narrowed pulse pressure can occur with both tampon-ade and tension pneumothorax.

▶ Lungs are clear BUT unequal in pneumothorax.

▶ Heart sounds are distant but hard to perceive in this setting.

Shock—Tension Pneumothorax

▶ Tension pneumothorax, also more commonly associated with trauma, can occur in medical situations, especially with positive pressure ventilation.

▶ This phenomenon is air or gas trapped in the pleural cavity. For example, a COPD patient ruptures a bleb (bubble on the lung surface) and progressive air trapping occurs.

▶ Clues/Differentials: (as with cardiac tamponade)

— Pulsus paradoxus

— Neck vein distension

— Narrowed pulse pressure

▶ Sudden dyspnea with pleuritic chest pain is common with ruptured bleb (along with increasing dyspnea and unequal lung sounds).

▶ Unequal lung sounds with increasing dyspnea is the key. Especially noteworthy is the fact that the unequal lung sounds on the affected side will have noticeable decrease with both inhalation and exhalation—very discriminating.

▶ Both phenomenon result in blue-gray skin around nose and mouth due to hypoxia.

Slide R-30   **Shock—Distributive**

▶ This is a transition slide used to introduce the next category of shock—distributive.

▶ This is a category of shock that results from vessel dilation or permeability (leaking) or both.

▶ The actual causes will be discussed individually with emphasis on how the signs and symptoms differ from "classic" hemorrhagic shock.

Slide R-31   **Shock—Neurogenic**

▶ Neurogenic shock occurs when preload and afterload drops (and subsequently cardiac output) with widespread vessel dilation from sympathetic nervous system (SNS) failure.

— Usually associated with traumatic spinal cord disease but some medical causes, such as septic toxins or poisons, may initiate this response.

— When some vessels dilate, the body usually compensates by constricting other vessels (shunt).

— With this type of shock, nearly all the vessels dilate at once.

— When due to poisons or toxins, the brainstem is affected and respiratory and cardiac effects also may be exhibited.

▶ Clues/Differentials: This type of shock *does not* resemble the classic signs of hemorrhagic shock.

— Skin vitals: warm, dry, and good tone. There may not be sweating.

— Initially, the patient may be hyperperfused, but as shock progresses:

▪ Blood pools in dependent parts and the upper surface of the body becomes pale and cool as the body loses heat.

▪ Heart rate is variable and depends on the toxin involved.

▶ Heroin, beta blockers, and insecticides interfere with the SNS and cause bradycardia.

— Respiratory rate will always be compromised.

— Pulmonary edema may occur.

Slide R-32   **Shock—Anaphylactic**

▶ Anaphylactic shock is a negative feedback, immune response that is exaggerated.

▶ The reaction severity and speed depends on the allergen, the route, and the history of previous exposures.

▶ Signs and symptoms depend upon the target organ susceptible to the histamine and other chemicals released by the surrounding mast cells.

▶ The response causes widespread vessel dilation and leaking.

▶ Clues/Differentials: Depends on the target organ—usually vascular, lungs, GI tract, or skin.
— Skin: General flushing and/or hives, itching, and swelling (especially in the mucous membranes); petechia may be evident.
— If the skin is not the target organ, general pallor and/or cyanosis may only be present.
— GI: Smooth muscles contraction with vasodilation and leaking in the GI tract (if the target organ) causes stomach cramps, vomiting, and protracted diarrhea.
— Respiratory: Smooth muscle contraction and permeability may cause bronchospasms (wheezing) and laryngospasm (stridor) or respiratory arrest.
— BP/pulse: Drop in cardiac output causes compensatory tachycardia.

Slide R-33   **Shock—Septic**
▶ Septic shock results from an overwhelming infection and may not be noticed for quite a while and may be confused with a variety of other problems.
▶ Begins with the infection itself and the systemic effect from the endotoxins, and the body's attempt to get rid of it—chills, fever, tachycardia (except in young children and the elderly), tachypnea (hypermetabolic stage).
▶ The specific signs and symptoms depend upon the underlying condition of the patient, the causative organism, and the organs involved.
▶ In the last stage, toxins have caused extreme vessel leaking with a drop in cardiac output and potential pulmonary edema.
▶ Clues/Differentials: Depends on age of patient and stage of sepsis.
— Skin:
  ▪ If hyperdynamic: flushed and pink (fever)
  ▪ If later stages: pallor and cyanosis
— Widespread microemboli with vessel leaking cause petechiae.
— Meningococcus creates a large purple or blue appearing spot called purpura (non-blanching). Other bacteria may cause skin peeling, especially over palmer surfaces of the hands and soles of feet.
▶ ALWAYS ASK if the patient has had a recent fever as part of the history gathering.
— Lungs: Usually a target organ so dyspnea and altered lung sounds are common (don't confuse this with CHF in the elderly).
— BP: Initially high with the hyperdynamic state, then falls late.
— Mental status: Due to hypoxia and the development of poor glucose use, the brain cells are affected.

Slide R-34 **Shock—Cardiogenic**
▶ Abnormal heart function of some type causes cardiogenic shock.
▶ Rhythm disturbances, poor muscle function, valve disorders, and acute MI with heart wall damage are the causes.
▶ Clues/Differentials:
— LISTENING TO LUNG SOUNDS is the key. The provider must differentiate this from other forms of shock as the treatment may be significantly different.
— Lung sounds: pulmonary edema with crackles, diminished lung sounds, and sometimes wheezes; cough with white or pink-tinged sputum and dyspnea
— Skin: cyanosis due to hypoxia and a drop in cardiac output

NOTE: To wrap up this review of the key signs and symptoms that differentiate the cause of shock—point out two key pieces of information:
▶ Listen to lung sounds in the initial assessment.
▶ Find the organ or organ system involved.

Slide R-35 **Case Study 1: History**
▶ Reintroduce this case to the participants as they've looked at numerous slides since the presentation of the case's scene size-up and initial assessment.
▶ Recap: This is a 64-year-old male with acute onset of dyspnea and hypotension who has clear lung sounds but who shows signs of shock.
▶ Paraphrase OPQRST history, then move on to the next slide.

Slide R-36 **Case Study 1: History**
▶ Paraphrase SAMPLE history. Ask for impression and differentials again.

Slide R-37 **Case Study 1**
▶ Additional information describes a patient in shock with a probable pulmonary embolus.
▶ The participants should have included in their list of differentials: AMI with cardiogenic shock, post-op hemorrhagic shock.

NOTE: The pulse oximeter reading should be discussed since the patient's BP may not be perfusing the distal fingers very well—that reading may not be accurate.

Slide R-38 **Case Study 1: Final Impression**
▶ Final impression, as discussed above with differentials.
▶ Pathophysiology should be discussed, referring to PE as a form of obstructive shock which limits preload to the left ventricle and creates hypoxia from V/Q mismatch with poor cardiac output.
▶ Treatment, other than oxygen, IV, and monitors, should include consideration of a fluid bolus to challenge preload.
— Discuss use of vasoactive agents that may help with cardiac output, unless participants are sure that this is NOT hemorrhagic shock.

▶ Remind the participants that the ongoing assessment must re-evaluate this unstable patient frequently with reconsideration of the treatment plan, based on the final impression and differentials.

▶ Close Case Study 1 and segue to next case study.

Slide R-39   **Case Study 2**
Title slide for Case Study 2

Slide R-40   **Case Study 2: Shortness of Breath**
▶ Paraphrase the information on the slide in an attempt to paint the picture of the scene for scene size-up.

Ask: *Any concerns about this scene?*
     Any resources needed at this time?
— Reinforced answers: Scene appears safe but additional lifting help may be needed due to space confinement. Those resources should be called for early as part of scene management.

NOTE: DO NOT switch to the next slide until the group has discussed these questions with appropriate guidance and encouragement.

Slide R-41   **Case Study 2: Shortness of Breath**
▶ Review this information as the participants read it.

Ask: *Is this patient stable or unstable?*
— The discussion should include the fact that this is a very sick-looking patient and the providers should immediately assess and resuscitate the ABCDs aggressively.

Ask: *What information would you like now?*
— How is the airway?
— How is the patient breathing? Resuscitation for each prior to moving on.

Slide R-42   **Case Study 2: Shortness of Breath**
▶ Airway needs to be addressed immediately—even before moving on to breathing assessment.

Ask: *How should you manage this airway?*
— Discuss patient position, head-tilt/chin-lift, and use of airway adjuncts—including suction. Reassess after any intervention to make sure air is moving and no secretions obstructing.

Ask: *What do you note with the breathing assessment and what should be done?*
— This patient appears to be in respiratory failure from an unknown cause.
— Discuss that use of positive pressure ventilation with supplemental oxygen. Use of 2-person bag-valve-mask ventilation or pocket mask would be best. Reassessment of adequate minute volume is important.

▸ Point out that this patient is maintaining his cardiac output SO FAR.

— He has an altered mental status with respiratory distress.

Ask: *Could this be from hypoxia? Or some other illness?*

— As the ABCDs are resuscitated, further information is necessary.

Ask: *What could cause an acute dyspneic episode in a patient who has signs of chronic disease (COPD)?*

— What else could be wrong?

— Is this respiratory distress or respiratory failure?

NOTE: Encourage discussion that includes the list of acute incidents that could trigger this type of patient situation.

▸ Segue to the next review slides that will be covering the possibilities . . .

Slide R-43   **Respiratory Failure**

▸ Assessment of a patient with a complaint of respiratory distress should include looking for signs of respiratory failure.

▸ This slide lists the signs and symptoms to watch for in trying to identify the patient who is decompensating and is threatening to arrest.

Slide R-44   **History in Dyspnea**

▸ When obtaining history, the provider should determine whether this incident came on suddenly or gradually— possibilities of what could be wrong can be ruled in and ruled out with this information (e.g., pneumonia vs. pulmonary edema).

▸ Ask participants which types of respiratory distress episodes would come on gradually vs. suddenly. Support the discussion.

NOTE: Each of the OPQRST history questions will not be reviewed here unless you wish to add information on:

▸ P: Fresh air, body position

▸ Q: Pain type (described)

— If sharp: pleural effusion, pneumothorax, or PE

— If tightness or squeeze: AMI, asthma

▸ R: (No special differentials)

▸ S: Severity is discussed on the next slide.

Slide R-45   **History in Dyspnea**

▸ In history gathering for the chronic respiratory patient, the provider should determine the severity of the dyspnea from the patient's point of view.

▸ The patient with chronic respiratory problems will have experience with his/her disease and the different levels of discomfort associated with it.

— Does it chronically interfere with life?

▸ During an acute exacerbation: The provider should determine severity via 0–10 scale, and if the number is high according to the patient, ask what happened the last time the dyspnea became this severe (e.g., the asthmatic who says 10 on the scale and indicates that the last time it was this bad, intubation occurred).

▶ Resting vs. exertional dyspnea indicates severity as well.

▶ Note whether the patient can speak in full sentences.

   — The provider may describe how severe to others involved by mentioning how many word sentences the dyspneic patient can speak (e.g., speaks in 2-word sentences).

NOTE: Time is not individually discussed on the slide as part of the OPQRST.

▶ Elicit discussion with the group in differentiating chronic vs. acute dyspnea or the chronically dyspneic patient who is having a sudden "episode" (similar to the patient in Case Study 2).

Slide R-46   **Differentials in Dyspnea**

▶ This slide reminds the participant to determine why this patient is dyspneic.

▶ Review this information with the participants and possibly relate it to Case Study 2.

Ask: *Which of these do you think is causing dyspnea in our patient?*

NOTE: This is a nice segue to differentials in the patient with difficulty breathing. The next few slides will review the differentials in the cause of dyspnea . . . first, we'll review airway obstruction.

Slide R-47   **Airway**

▶ Airway obstruction as a potential cause of dyspnea usually develops suddenly.

▶ If foreign body:

   — Is there evidence of recent ingestion?

   — Can you see the foreign body in the pharynx?

   — REMEMBER: The most common cause of airway obstruction is FBAO in the conscious patient.

▶ If infection of pharynx or upper airway:

   — Any fever?

   — Dysphagia?

   — Trismus?

   — Any symptoms of epiglottitis?

   — Ludwig's angina?

   — Retropharyngeal abscess?

▶ If anaphylaxis:

   — Any symptoms of sudden onset, allergic reaction?

   — Any recent sting, ingestion, injection, etc.?

▶ Angioedema develops suddenly in those with hereditary tendency during times of stress, trauma, or surgery.

   — A newer drug category: ACE inhibitors have been implicated in angioedema too.

▶ Other causes of airway obstruction: hematoma for those on platelet inhibiting drugs

Slide R-48   Respiratory Causes of Dyspnea

▶ As a differential in the patient with dyspnea, the respiratory system itself could be the culprit.

▶ Asthma: This disease is not diagnosed by the physician overnight. It usually takes several wheezing or coughing episodes in the patient's life to appropriately diagnose the ailment.

— It can develop in any age group.

— There must be a history of asthma or the patient states, "I think it's asthma." Asthma attacks are sudden in onset. There will be inhalers prescribed and the history of their use may be key in understanding the severity of the disease and how bad this attack is.

— The respirations have a prolonged expiratory phase and wheezing may or may not be apparent (if not enough air moving—no wheezing).

— Most asthma patients have a very good understanding of how to chronically control their disease and how to resuscitate their own attacks to a certain point.

▶ COPD: This is another chronic respiratory disease with occasional, acute exacerbations. It is further classified into chronic bronchitis and emphysema.

— Chronic bronchitis patients tend to be somewhat obese and have a chronic low oxygen saturation and chronic productive cough.

— Emphysema patients are generally thin with a large barrel chest and distant lung sounds.

— Most COPD patients have elements of both chronic bronchitis and emphysema. Acute episodes are characterized by cough, wheeze, and sputum production (always ask the color).

— Exacerbations are usually due to poor medication compliance, weather changes, infections, environmental exposures, and certain sedative-like medications.

▶ If you find the patient within his/her own home, there is usually evidence of home-care equipment and probably inhalers.

Slide R-49   Additional Respiratory Causes of Dyspnea

▶ The following conditions are gradual onsets of dyspnea:

— Pneumonia is either bacterial or non-bacterial in nature and if chronic diseases are present (CNS), there is a possibility of aspiration pneumonia.

▪ General signs of being "sick" are present with complaints of chills, fever, malaise, aches, pleuritic chest pain, and dyspnea.

— Pleural effusion: also presents in a gradual way, depending upon the underlying disease (renal failure, pancreatitis, infection, PE, liver disease, CHF, etc.) with diminished lung sounds and a complaint of pleuritic chest pain.

— Pleurytis/pleurodynia: an inflammatory condition of the chest wall. Pleuritic chest pain without fever and an occasional pleural friction rub auscultated.

Slide R-50   **Additional Respiratory Causes of Dyspnea**

▶ These two conditions, as described in Case Study 1, have a sudden onset of symptoms:

— Pneumothorax and tension pneumothorax: Can occur in young patients, especially tall, thin-bodied males. Asthma, pneumonia, COPD can develop pneumothoraces.

▪ REMEMBER that most medical pneumothoraces occur because of positive pressure ventilation.

▪ Usually a sudden onset of pleuritic pain after strain or cough

— Pulmonary embolus: arterial blockage of the pulmonary circulation, creating a diminished preload to the left ventricle (obstructive shock) if large enough.

▪ The provider should delve into the common risk factors for the development of PE (e.g., recent immobility, recent surgery or travel, birth control pills, or hereditary coagulation disorders).

▪ Dyspnea, pleuritic chest pain (at times), and cough are symptoms. Tachycardia and tachypnea are common. Secondary findings, such as a change in lung sounds, tenderness in an extremity (DVT), or changes in a 12-lead ECG are more rare.

Slide R-51   **Cardiac Causes of Dyspnea**

▶ In order to develop our impression and differentials, consider the cardiac causes of dyspnea.

— Remember that some patients do not present with classic chest pain while suffering from AMI. Certain patient populations, such as diabetics, the elderly, and those with chronic hypertension, may present with acute breathlessness. Nausea, sweating, fatigue, and vertigo may also be present. Any patient complaining of an acute onset of dyspnea must have AMI ruled out.

— Those with chronic ischemic heart disease may not have any signs. But if they do, crackles may be heard in the lung bases (left heart failure); a soft first heart sound, split second heart sound, or gallop rhythms are very difficult to appreciate in the prehospital setting, but may be found.

— Congestive heart failure may be a chronic disease under control with medications and other outpatient therapy. Occasionally, these patients develop an acute exacerbation with increased dyspnea, increased work of breathing, orthopnea, paroxysmal nocturnal dyspnea (PND), occasional wheezing (cardiac asthma), but classic signs include crackles in the bases with occasional extremity edema and JVD.

— EXTREME CAUTION must be exercised when dealing with older patients who may be wheezing in CHF as they may also have components of COPD.

— Cardiac tamponade is usually a life-threatening condition, seen as a result of pericarditis from infection, or in patients with renal failure, cancer, drug abuse, and diseases such as lupus. Dyspnea, orthopnea, and paroxysmal nocturnal dyspnea are major symptoms. There may be JVD, hepatomegaly, pericardial friction rub, and pulsus paradoxus.

Slide R-52   **Dyspnea/CNS**

▶ The sensation of dyspnea may occur in CNS disorders due to weakened respiratory muscles, especially if complicated by infection, pneumonia, or other stressors.

— Amyotrophic lateral sclerosis (ALS, Lou Gehrig's disease) presents with chronic and progressive muscle wasting with intact mental function. Swallowing, respiratory muscles, speech, and proximal muscles are affected.

— Guillain-Barré presents with weakness that progresses in an opposite order than expected—distal to proximal—and may affect respiratory muscles. This disorder typically is preceded by a viral illness.

— Myasthenia gravis affects the motor endplates and appears worse with exertion and improves when the patient rests. This disease also may affect respiratory muscles and typically includes visual changes.

Slide R-53   **Dyspnea/Other**

▶ This is the last of the slides that differentiates the causes of dyspnea.

— Anemia creates a pale patient who becomes tachycardic and tachypneic quite easily, especially with exertion, and if severe, position changes (hemorrhagic shock). Dyspnea is due to the fact that there isn't enough hemoglobin to deliver oxygen. Severe anemia may lead to CHF.

— Hyperthyroidism: The body's increased metabolic demands create a need for more respiratory drive, thus dyspnea. These patients appear thin, oily, and have hair loss. They may be nervous, have tremors, and chronic diarrhea.

— Metabolic acidosis: A variety of causes such as infection, renal failure, drug overdoses, and diabetes may create a metabolic acidosis that presents with tachypnea/hyperpnea and a feeling of dyspnea with clear lung sounds.

— Psychogenic hyperventilation: Created by psychological stress and is diagnosed ONLY after all other causes have been eliminated and not in the prehospital setting.

NOTE: Remind the participants of what the patient in Case Study 2 has shown us so far . . . An older gentleman with a barrel chest rushes in from the street and is found leaning against a wall and appears to be in potential respiratory failure. We've been attempting to define what our initial list of differentials should be in this case.

Slide R-54   **Case Study 2**
▶ Allow only the top information on the slide to appear first.

Ask: *How should we now treat this patient who looks as though he is in respiratory failure?*
— Discussion should be encouraged but emergency treatment includes positioning the patient appropriately and delivering positive pressure ventilation (PPV) with oxygen (when available).
▶ The next section of the slide can then appear to show that BVM has been attempted and the patient's chest won't rise.

Ask: *What is wrong and what should we do to correct this?*
▶ Encourage discussion before moving to the next slide.
— 1st: Reposition patient's head/neck for airway and retry PPV.
— 2nd: If still no chest rise, attempt foreign body airway obstruction (FBAO) techniques, according to American Heart Association Guidelines (2000).
— If abdominal thrusts are not successful, the advanced provider should visualize the mid-airway with laryngoscope blade, use the Magill forceps, and remove any visible debris in the airway.

Slide R-55   **Case Study 2**
▶ This slide provides additional information that may help the participants if they still have mixed ideas on a final impression/differentials.
▶ Paraphrase this information as the participants read it.

Re-ask: *What is wrong with this patient?*
▶ The next slide asks for the final impression, differentials.

Slide R-56   **Case Study 2**
▶ The participants should discuss the pathophysiology and then develop a treatment plan for this patient.
— For instance: If they reposition this patient's airway and still cannot get the chest to rise with BVM, they should attempt basic FBAO maneuvers (5 abdominal thrusts with finger sweeps) as they acquire Magill forceps and intubation equipment in order to attempt a direct visualization of the airway.
— A surgical airway may be discussed but participants must include information on determining where the obstruction is vs. the artificial airway site and whether that dramatic procedure would work.

NOTE: This is the end of Case Study 2. Have participants take a 15-minute break and then come back to complete Part II of the AMLS Refresher review.

SLIDE NO.   **SLIDE TITLE/NOTES**

Slide R-57   **AMLS Refresher Review—Part II**
There will be three more cases discussed by the participants, led and encouraged by the instructor.

Slide R-58   **Case Study 3: Abdominal Pain**
Title slide for Case Study 3. This case setting is in an emergency department.

Slide R-59   **Case Study 3**
▶ Paraphrase this information as the participants read through it.

Ask: *Is this patient stable or unstable? (At a triage desk, should this patient go to the waiting room, wait in a side room, or be given a higher priority for entrance in the ED proper?)*
▶ Guide and encourage discussion. Some providers with experience in the ED setting may veer to regional/local problems with busy EDs.
▶ Our task is to guide the discussion to determine whether (in a perfect world) this patient might be given a higher priority than a patient with a laceration, for instance.
▶ Reinforce discussion: ABCD are intact, but acute abdominal pain indicates a red flag.
▶ A differential diagnosis determined in the field takes on a far different meaning than in the hospital setting. EMS usually determines if this is a life-threatening, potential life-threatening, or non-life-threatening situation. In the hospital setting, a great deal of time is usually taken to determine the cause of acute abdominal pain.

Slide R-60   **Case Study 3**
▶ This slide is intended to answer the question on the previous slide.

Slide R-61   **Case Study 3**
▶ This slide reviews the initial assessment completed in a triage area and provides some guidance as to the priority of the patient.
▶ Quiet tachypnea, or a fast respiratory rate without use of accessory muscles, may indicate an acidotic state, shock, or other conditions that warrant attention.

Ask: *Is this patient stable or unstable?*
What initial treatment or assessments need to be applied?
▶ Encourage discussion. This is a stable patient with an acute problem. Monitors, lab analysis, IV, and other diagnostics may be included in the discussion.

	SLIDE NO.	SLIDE TITLE/NOTES

Slide R-62   **Case Study 3**
- ▶ This slide reviews the initial treatment applied and diagnostics ordered and may be reviewed (without reciting).

Ask: *Initial Impression?*
    Differentials?
- ▶ Lead and encourage discussion.
  - — Reinforced possibilities include: appendicitis, diverticulitis, cholecystitis, AMI, pneumonia, aortic disruption, gastritis, peptic ulcer disease (PUD).
- ▶ The next two slides will discuss the OPQRST and SAMPLE history of this case.

Slide R-63   **Case Study 3**
- ▶ OPQRST history reviewed.

Ask: *What is your initial impression given this information?*
    Differentials?
- — The same list of possibilities may be discussed as in slide R-62.

Slide R-64   **Case Study 3**
- ▶ SAMPLE history reviewed.
- ▶ Repeat above questions with same possibilities discussed.

Slide R-65   **Case Study 3**
- ▶ Focused exam reveals a clinically negative abdomen and the surprise information of an undiagnosed hyperglycemic patient.

Ask: *What could cause epigastric discomfort and dyspnea in a patient with diabetes?*
- ▶ Review the differentials in determining the cause of abdominal pain in an attempt to answer the above question.

Slide R-66   **Referred Pain**
- ▶ Spleen: close to the diaphragm and left phrenic nerve, thereby referred to the left neck and shoulder
- ▶ Ovary/fallopian tubes: ruptured capsules release chemical of inflammation to the peritoneal lining, diaphragm, and phrenic nerves, thereby referred to either side of the neck or shoulders
- ▶ The heart sits in the dome of the diaphragm so epigastric pain common and vagal stimulation creates the associated nausea and vomiting.
- ▶ Appendicitis (early) creates visceral, poorly localized pain that may be peri-umbilical or epigastric.
- ▶ Diverticulitis may cause the same type of poorly localized pain.
- ▶ Appendicitis pain can be located in the epigastric/umbilical area.
- ▶ Kidney stone pain may refer to the groin from the flank.

Slide R-67   **Referred Pain**

▶ Liver: Because of its proximity to the diaphragm, disease of the liver can cause referred pain along the phrenic nerve to the right neck and shoulder.

▶ Gallbladder: Due to its location, if disease is localized at the gallbladder or hepatic duct, pain will be referred to the right scapula or between the scapulae.

▶ Pancreas: The location of the pancreas is beneath the stomach and extends into the curve of the duodenum and the spleen. It is both a peritoneal and retroperitoneal organ so pain is many times in the mid back.

▶ Abdominal aorta: Within the retroperitoneal space, pain from a tear in this structure may create a visceral pain in the lumbosacral area with radiation to the front—abdomen and anterior legs.

Slide R-68   **Extra-Abdominal Causes of Abdominal Pain**

▶ The extra-abdominal causes of abdominal pain are listed by symptoms and differential diagnoses. This slide is also intended to pinpoint the cause of abdominal pain in Case Study 3.

— AMI may create diffuse abdominal pain and indigestion perceived as pain.

— Pneumonia may lead to diffuse abdominal pain with no local tenderness but cough and fever accompany the complaint.

— DKA: With high K+ levels, abdominal smooth muscles may cramp.

— Drug withdrawal creates a severe colicky pain.

— Sickle cell disease may cause severe abdominal pain due to splenic infarction.

— Spinal or CNS illness can cause pain referred to the abdomen.

▶ Refer to sources of abdominal pain by region as per slides R-69 to R-75.

Slide R-69   **Right Hypochondriac**

▶ Liver: steady, dull with radiation to right neck and shoulder from hepatitis, cirrhosis, with resulting ascites which may cause dyspnea, distended abdomen

▶ Gallbladder: tucked under the right lobe of the liver, typical RUQ pain with referral to right scapula or between the scapulae if stones

▶ Referred pain to this area can come from pleuritis, pneumonia on right.

Slide R-70   **Epigastric**

▶ Stomach: located primarily in the epigastric region with possibilities of referred pain into left or right hypochondriac regions from gastritis

▶ Pancreas: a 20-cm long organ behind the stomach and extends from the duodenum to the spleen; epigastric pain, bores into the back (retro).

▶ Referred pain to the epigastric region comes from AMI or appendicitis.

Slide R-71 Left Hypochondriac

▶ Spleen: located on the left behind the stomach and beneath diaphragm; creates steady and dull pain with referral to the left shoulder and neck

▶ Pancreas: as described in the previous slide; next to the spleen

▶ Referred pain to this area is usually from pleuritis or pneumonia.

Slide R-72 Central Abdomen

▶ Small intestine: intermittent, crampy or colicky dull pain

▶ Large intestine: from just beneath the stomach/liver and frames the small bowel

▶ Aorta: a retroperitoneal organ creates visceral pain in lumbar-sacral back/abdomen

▶ Referred pain to this region is usually due to large bowel obstruction.

Slide R-73 Lumbar

▶ Kidneys/ureters: Kidneys are located in the retroperitoneal space with dull and steady pain on posterior affected side. Ureters create colicky pain that many times refers to the groin.

Slide R-74 Right Iliac

▶ Appendix: Early inflammation can create periumbilical or epigastric pain but as it progresses, localizes to McBurney's point.

▶ Ovaries/fallopian tubes: Dull, constant pain in affected side is typical of ovarian problems. Fallopian tube pain is colicky and intermittent on affected side.

Slide R-75 Left Iliac

▶ Large intestine: as described earlier, mostly referred to the umbilical or hypogastric region

▶ Left ovary and tube: as described in the previous slide

NOTE: Recap Case Study 3: Middle-aged gentleman who thinks of himself as healthy developed epigastric pain with dyspnea two days ago. His abdomen is negative to exam. Apparently newly diagnosed diabetes. In the ED with oxygen, IV, and a cardiac monitor on. Diagnostics being performed. Attempting to find the cause of his complaints.

Slide R-76 Case Study 3

▶ Review this information with the participants as they discover that this patient is suffering from an AMI.

▶ Discuss the pathophysiology with participants and give guidance and encouragement.

▶ New, undiagnosed diabetics in their adult years many times present in two ways to the healthcare system: AMI or DKA.

▶ The patient may have been suffering from hyperglycemia for quite a while.

▶ The vascular disease has created an ischemic cascade of his heart muscle, but pain is not well localized by the diabetic.

▶ A combination of epigastric discomfort with dyspnea should be considered AMI until proven otherwise.

▶ This patient will need to be worked up for either mechanical or chemical clot intervention in the right coronary artery and for his diabetes.

Slide R-77   **Case Study 4: Chest Pain**
Title slide for Case Study 4

Slide R-78   **Case Study 4**

▶ EMS is responding to a remote dialysis unit for a patient complaining of chest pain. Ask the participants to size up the scene, and from the doorway, determine if the patient appears to be stable or unstable (until more assessment can be done).

Slide R-79   **Case Study 4**

▶ As you arrive at the side of the patient, the dialysis nurse describes the situation and you assess the ABCDs.

▶ Repeat the question about stability.

Ask: *Initial management?*
       What assessment needs to be acquired?
— Oxygen, IV, and cardiac monitor with 12-lead ECG (if available); history and focused assessment

Slide R-80   **Case Study 4**

▶ Review the initial assessment information and history.

NOTE: Wait until the 3rd slide in this series prior to asking for initial impression vs. differentials.

Slide R-81   **Case Study 4**

▶ History shows a 2-day history of non-radiating pain that worsens when the patient lays down.

Slide R-82   **Case Study 4**

▶ SAMPLE history confirms the past medical history of diabetes with renal failure that is treated with dialysis and the recent history of a late dialysis run.

Ask: *Initial Impression?*
      Differentials?
▶ With subsequent discussion by the participants, the possibilities might include: AMI, tamponade, tension pneumothorax, aortic dissection, pneumonia, PE, intra-abdominal causes such as PUD, gastritis, esophageal tear, cholecystitis, pleurodynia, costochrondritis, etc.

▶ Review differentials in identification of the cause of chest pain.

	SLIDE NO.	SLIDE TITLE/NOTES

Slide R-83 **Chest Pain**
- ▶ This is a generic statement that segues the discussion to differentials in chest pain.

Ask: *Is this cardiac chest pain?*
- — A major possibility.
- ▶ This is important as treatment can be carried out in the field, and time is significant to overall survival.

NOTE: The table slides can be a bit confusing. It is important to highlight key points for participants.

Slide R-84 **AMI**
- ▶ AMI should be suspected in males over 30 and females over 40, especially with positive risk factors for this disease.
- ▶ Review classic signs and symptoms and then highlight that diabetics and females sometimes present without chest pain.
- ▶ Associated symptoms highlighted:
  - — Physical findings are usually not helpful in the diagnosis.
  - — An early 12-lead ECG needs to be done but not relied upon as THE diagnostic in identification of AMI, as a normal ECG can be seen in many ischemic cascades.
  - — Standard treatment includes oxygen, IV, and monitor(s), with aspirin early, along with vasoactive, pain management.

Slide R-85 **Aortic Dissection**
- ▶ Aortic dissection is fairly rare and hard to differentiate in the prehospital setting. The classic patient is a hypertensive male of 40–70 years of age.
- ▶ A tear in the intimal layer of the artery creates an artificial ballooning of the vessel (aneurysm) with pain that reflects the pathophysiology—tearing pain that is severe at first, then becomes intermittent. Depending on location of the dissection, symptoms vary:
  - — Aortic arch: Carotid and subclavian involvement creates stroke-like symptoms or a pulseless arm. If it is extensive, it creates cardiac tamponade.
  - — Descending thoracic/abdominal/iliac aorta: These dissections traverse into the arteries that perfuse individual organs at times. For instance, iliac dissection may progress to the renal artery and symptoms might include hematuria.
- ▶ Depending on location and symptoms, treatment may be either medical or surgical.
- ▶ Ehlers-Danlos syndrome: Inherited disorder of connective tissue that makes the vessels fragile. Aortic dissection may occur in younger patients with this disorder.
- ▶ Marfan's syndrome: Hereditary disorder of connective tissue that creates a tall, lean body with long extremities (fingers and toes). Aorta is dilated and susceptible to dissection.

Slide R-86   **Pulmonary Embolism**

▶ Pulmonary embolism (discussed in earlier case as obstructive shock) may produce chest pain. If greater than half of the pulmonary vasculature is involved, this is a serious, life-threatening condition with shock symptoms, dyspnea, and hypoxia.

▶ Symptoms may be described as sharp, pleuritic chest pain, tachycardia, and tachypnea. Physical findings not usually helpful but lung sounds may include crackles, pleural rub.

▶ Discuss the risk factors associated with 80% of PEs.

Slide R-87   **Esophageal**

▶ Perforation of the esophagus occurs with sudden, forceful rise in the intra-abdominal or intrathoracic pressures (e.g., forceful vomiting, coughing, or post-procedures such as endoscopic exam).

▶ GI contents leak into the mediastinum—overwhelming infection will occur, but chest pain is first. Chest pain is sharp, steady in the anterior, posterior, and epigastric regions. May radiate to the neck. Associated symptoms include dysphagia and hemoptysis with pleural friction rub, tachycardia, tachypnea, hypotension.

▶ Treatment is geared to supporting the septic patient with monitors, oxygen, fluids, and transport to a cardiothoracic surgeon.

Slide R-88   **Cardiac Tamponade**

▶ Cardiac tamponade develops in a medical setting via accumulation of fluids into the pericardial sac. This fills to the point of compromising cardiac filling and drops cardiac output—thus shock.

— If from an infectious condition like pericarditis, chest pain may be present.

▶ Malignant pericardial effusion does not usually presents with chest pain. Symptoms similar to pericarditis—positional chest pain. Renal failure patients who accumulate fluid tend to create pericardial and pleural effusions also.

▶ If tamponade, Beck's Triad apparent.

Slide R-89   **Tension Pneumothorax**

▶ Tension pneumothorax, as a cause of chest pain, has been discussed earlier in the obstructive shock portion of this review.

▶ Tension pneumothorax in a medical setting usually occurs with congenital or acquired weakened thoracic tissue, creating a spontaneous pneumothorax that progresses. This can also occur in COPD patients, those with cancer of lung tissue, or lung infections and is rare in those who breathe on their own.

— This phenomenon occurs with much more frequency during positive pressure ventilation, especially with co-existing lung disease.

▶ If chest pain occurs, it is sudden and sharp, pleuritic in nature, and accompanied by tachypnea, dyspnea, tachycardia, with splinted respirations.

Slide R-90   **Pericarditis**

▶ An inflammatory condition that produces steady, burning, retrosternal chest pain that may radiate into the back, neck, scapula, or jaw. It may worsen with deep breath and pulsate with each beat of the heart. It is worse upon lying down—improves with sitting up or leaning forward (positional chest pain).

▶ A pericardial rub might be heard if conditions were silent in the environment and the healthcare provider was trained to auscultate this abnormal heart sound. There may be ST-segment elevation or depression throughout leads, without localization.

Slide R-91   **Costochondritis**

▶ Inflammation of the ribs and cartilage supporting the ribs may develop after an upper respiratory infection. The chest pain is usually sharp and made worse by chest-wall and arm movement.

▶ There may be point tenderness at the site upon palpation of the chest wall. *But* patients suffering AMI and PE may also have point tenderness, *so* costochondritis should never be diagnosed in the field.

Slide R-92   **Pleurdynia**

▶ Inflammatory condition of the parietal pleura with sharp, pleuritic pain and few other symptoms

▶ No or few physical findings, possibly a pleural friction rub; similar to costochondritis

Slide R-93   **GI Disorders**

▶ GI disorders can cause chest pain too.

▶ Peptic ulcer disease (PUD), acute cholecystitis, esophagitis, esophageal spasm, and gastroesophageal reflux (GERD) are some conditions that may cause this.
— Sensory nerve fibers are shared between many abdominal structures and the thorax.

▶ Usually retrosternal burning, similar to AMI. May radiate to the throat and cause heartburn. Worse at night, especially when lying supine or leaning far forward.

▶ Esophageal spasm is just like an AMI in appearance and usually improves with administration of nitroglycerin. (Conversely, AMI pain can be relieved with antacids.)

Slide R-94   **Mitral Valve**

▶ Elastic mitral valve expands into the left atrium during systole and can create episodes of chest pain due to stretching of the chordae tendinae and papillary muscles.

▶ Associated symptoms include vertigo, dyspnea, palpitations, and syncope.

▶ Systolic murmur (click) and cardiac dysrhythmias may be found. Most patients with this condition are asymptomatic.

NOTE: Recap Case Study 4: Older diabetic female who is a day and a half late for a dialysis run, complaining of positional chest pain (worse lying down) that does not radiate.

Slide R-95 **Case Study 4**

▶ Review assessment findings (once history obtained) with the participants.

▶ 12-lead ECG not that helpful in that LBBB is present which distorts ST-segment (without comparison with previous ECGs).

▶ The patient shows signs of elevated right heart pressure (JVD) and has distal and proximal edema. Pulsus paradoxus sign is present.

▶ The next slide will ask for final impression.

Slide R-96 **Case Study 4**

▶ Final impression should be pericardial effusion, creating tamponade. These chronic effusions may have hundreds of cc's of fluid that would never be tolerated by the patient. An acute accumulation of 50–100 cc is adaptable when slow filling occurs. If not drained, cardiac output will drop to the point of cardiac arrest in a pulseless electrical activity presentation.

Slide R-97 **Case Study 5: Altered Mental Status**
Title slide for Case Study 5

Slide R-98 **Case Study 5**

▶ This descriptive slide attempts to paint a picture of a hot, summer day at a fairgrounds. The case shows a female waving the EMS crew to her trailer for a man who she describes as being "altered" (ain't right).
— Guide discussion on this scene size-up. Patients with altered mental status may be very difficult to handle.

Ask: *Should they call for additional resources now?*
— The simple answer is "yes."

Slide R-99 **Case Study 5**

▶ As they arrive, additional information is obtained that should make the participants want to immediately back out of the trailer. Unsafe!

▶ Additional resources are needed quickly as any patient with an altered mental status is considered unstable.

▶ Encourage discussion about what resources may be requested, how long they should wait, etc.

Slide R-100 **Case Study 5**

▶ As the crew waits outside the trailer for help, the female caller adds more information: The patient was OK two hours ago but not "feeling well," and she found the patient five minutes ago in this condition. She appears quite anxious and concerned, reinforcing the fact that this is a unique situation for the patient.

Slide R-101   **Case Study 5**
▶ Review ABCD exam information on this slide and, from the information so far . . .

Ask: *Is the patient stable or unstable?*
— This has pretty much been answered—unstable.

Ask: *Immediate treatment needed?*
— In most situations with an unstable patient, the health-care providers should immediately attempt to resuscitate whatever has been found wrong in the ABCD mnemonic. In this case—if lucky—may be able to apply oxygen, place monitor(s), and start an IV as further exam and history is gathered.

Slide R-102   **Case Study 5**
▶ The officers and helpers perform a safe take down on this patient.
▶ Discuss take-down techniques.
▶ The patient's skin is too hot and moist to keep patches on— even if he didn't take them off. He also removes the oxygen appliance from his face.
▶ Due to his continuous movement and agitation, an IV is not attempted in this situation.

Slide R-103   **Case Study 5**
▶ In this and the next slide, further history is obtained once the patient is safely secured in the EMS truck. Review the information without reading it to the participants.

Ask: *What could be wrong with a patient with a sudden onset of altered mental status who may have a fever?*
— The possibilities might include an intracerebral infection, tumor, toxins, environmental extremes, exacerbation of a chronic condition (diabetes), etc.

Slide R-104   **Case Study 5**
▶ This is the SAMPLE history. Lead the same discussion with encouragement on initial impression and differentials.
▶ On this slide, a recent ear infection should be emphasized, along with 5 hours since last intake of food. Remind everyone of the hot day.

NOTE: The table slides can be a bit confusing. It is important to highlight key points for participants.
▶ Review the differentials to consider when taking care of a patient with altered mental status. Focus on key information within the slides that makes that affliction's presentation or symptoms "different."

Slide R-105 **Environmental Clues**

▶ Clues from the environment that could help with differentials in AMS

— Temperature factors: chief complaint of confusion, delirium, AMS with accompanying signs of dehydration (cold and hot), respiratory compromise and tachycardias/bradycardias with altered perfusion. Very slow respirations accompany hypothermia and the end of heat stroke; tachypnea occurs with heat exhaustion, early heat stroke.

— Warm to hot skin (with or without sweating) in any heat emergency

— History of chronic conditions that may alter the patient's ability to sense extremes in temperature (diabetes, alcohol, drugs, poor circulation)

— Poor living conditions (chronic) with syringes, alcohol bottles in evidence

▪ May indicate electrolyte disturbances, Wernicke's or Korsakoff's, overdose

Slide R-106 **Clinical Findings**

▶ Extremes of blood sugar may lead to the appropriate impression.

▶ All altered mental status patients should have blood glucose assessment although further history on onset of action is key.

▶ Cardiac disorders with dysrhythmias and resulting drop in cardiac output may alter the mental status, along with the electrolyte disturbances that accompany poor perfusion and its treatment.

Slide R-107 **Behavior Clues**

▶ Bizarre behavior may be a clue to seizure, stroke, cranial infections, tumor, and other diseases listed on the slide. Find out if the patient has had a recent infection, fever and if the condition came on suddenly or slowly.

▶ The 2nd paragraph includes lassitude and confusion which may be caused by the conditions listed. Determining current chronic conditions (liver, diabetes, etc.) and onset of symptoms are key.

▶ The 3rd paragraph refers to a hyperdynamic state, possibly indicating thyroid disorders. Patients with hyperthyroidism usually have dry skin, small stature, prominent eyes, and tachycardias. Some drug overdoses also will create this behavior.

Slide R-108 **Miscellaneous Findings**

▶ AV shunt indicates renal failure and the AMS could be due to uremic encephalopathy, which also include nausea, vomiting, cramping, neuromuscular disorders, malaise, and Kussmaul's respirations (acidosis).

▶ Signs of diabetes are many times seen on the patient's body: Med Alert ID tags, signs of insulin administration (injection sites and syringes, insulin in the refrigerator), sores on the skin that look as though they are slow to heal, poor peripheral perfusion, signs of past amputations, scarring of the pads of the fingers from repeated glucose testing, and poor skin turgor.

▶ Clues on the body that can help you differentiate include looking for edema. Diseases that lead to body edema include CHF, cardiac failure, renal failure, electrolyte disturbances, and hypothyroidism (accompanied by larger body mass, oily skin, and loss of hair).

▶ The "polys" include eating too much (with weight loss), drinking too much, and urinating large amounts frequently. These are classic signs of high blood sugar from either undiagnosed or uncontrolled diabetes.

▶ If the patient complains of visual disturbances with altered mental status, this might lead you to think of intracranial vascular or infectious processes and electrolyte disturbances.

Slide R-109   Motor Symptoms

▶ Motor function that becomes uncoordinated, ataxic, etc. may be from the diseases listed in paragraph 1 of this slide. The brain is susceptible to small changes in pH, oxygenation, and glucose levels.

▶ Neurologic posturing of decerebration (extension) and decortication (flexion) can be caused by intracranial events such as tumor or stroke.

Slide R-110   Pain

▶ If a complaint of chest pain accompanies an altered mental status, the patient may be suffering from the items listed in paragraph 1 of this slide.

▶ We've referred to the sensitivity of the brain to small changes in pH, glucose, and oxygen, but narrow ranges of electrolyte imbalance can affect the CNS as well.

▶ Thyroid dysfunction can create chest pain, along with either hyperactive or hypoactive AMS.

▶ Toxins can alter the mental status and create chest pain.

▶ Extremes in temperature have been discussed.

▶ Neck pain and/or rigidity is usually associated with irritation/inflammation of the meninges that extend from the covering of the brain to the lumbar area of the spinal cord. Rash, fever, malaise, and other signs of sepsis would be present with this finding of pain.

Slide R-111   Skin Vitals

▶ Findings during AMS assessment of the patient's skin might give clues:
— Diaphoresis can indicate diabetic problems such as hypoglycemia as well as a heat emergency (exhaustion and stroke). Remember that those exercising in extreme heat can be sweaty as they enter the heat stroke phase.
— Fever indicates a hyperdynamic state—either from sepsis or hyperthyroidism. Heat emergencies may create this as well.

— Jaundice indicates poor circulation of bile and usually leads to thinking about possible liver disease. The liver may not be able to regulate ammonia levels and this leads to AMS. In addition to jaundice and AMS, these patients have a classic large belly (ascites), body edema, spider angiomas (spidery varicose veins), and fector hepaticus (musty odor to the breath).

— Poor skin turgor, sunken eyes, dry mucous membranes lead to thoughts of dehydration which could come with heat emergencies, hyperglycemia, and acute GI problems.

Slide R-112   Facial Symptoms

▶ When a patient with altered mental status has facial symptoms and dysphagia, this usually indicates hemiparesis from intracranial causes, but electrolyte disturbances (muscle control) and rising intracranial pressure from edema in liver failure could also create this affect.

Slide R-113   Drugs

▶ Clues that drugs may be a factor in the patient's altered mental status are listed here.

— Open bottles and drug paraphernalia might lead the healthcare worker to the impression of an overdose, toxic reaction, or metabolic acidosis/alkalosis with AMS.

— Syringes:
  ▪ Insulin: diabetes
  ▪ Tuberculin or larger syringes: toxic overdose

— Injection sites (same as above)

Slide R-114   Breathing

▶ Breathing patterns may indicate the underlying disease process:

— Kussmaul's: acidosis (deep, rapid)

— Central neurogenic: increased intracranial pressure (deep, rapid)

— Cheyne-Stokes: metabolic disease, stroke (pattern of irregularity)

— Biot's/Ataxic: stroke (uncoordinated)

— Apneustic: CNS disease, stroke (long, deep breaths with apnea)

— Abnormal breath odors:
  ▪ Fruity/ketones: hyperglycemia, DKA
  ▪ Musty: liver failure, hepatic encephalopathy

NOTE: Recap Case Study 5 as participants go back to figure out initial impression and differentials: This is a middle-aged male with a sudden onset of bizarre behavior in a hot environment. He seems to have a recent infection and is hard to control.

SLIDE NO.	SLIDE TITLE/NOTES

Slide R-115   **Case Study 5**
▶ Review the information with the participants.

Ask: *What is the Glasgow Coma score?*
— The score is 8.
▶ Point out the current fever—discuss whether muscle activity might have brought on this high fever or if the cause is an infection or environmental.
▶ Point out the general hyperdynamic state of this moving patient.

NOTE: The next slide will ask for final impression, differentials, and pathophysiology.

Slide R-116   **Case Study 5**
▶ The participants should have discussed hyperthermia secondary to a heat emergency (stroke) vs. intracranial infection vs. drug overdose with a hyperdynamic agent (methamphetamine, cocaine, etc.), vs. tumor with seizure.
▶ With the recent ear infection and fever, cranial abscess was found.
▶ In order to obtain diagnostic assessment and to control AMS and fever, rapid sequence induction for intubation was performed successfully.

Slide R-117   **Summary**
▶ This has been intended to be a review of the five major topics of AMLS: Hypoperfusion, Dyspnea, Abdominal Pain, Chest Pain, and Altered Mental Status via a case study format. The course will proceed to review the pretest questions and then group/team testing of these five topics and the written exam.

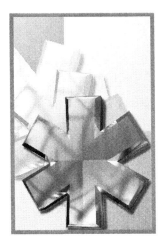

VI. ADVANCED MEDICAL LIFE SUPPORT COURSE ADMINISTRATION

⊞ AMLS MISSION STATEMENTS

The mission of the Advanced Medical Life Support (AMLS) programs is to compliment the National Association of Emergency Medical Technicians' mission by providing quality provider, instructor, and refresher programs that enhance the knowledge and skills of healthcare providers who care for patients experiencing a variety of medical emergencies. To that end, AMLS will provide healthcare providers the opportunity to participate in case-based interactive presentations and hands-on experiences that utilize comprehensive assessment and history taking skills, focused physical examinations, and formulation and progression from an initial or field impression to differential diagnosis and appropriate management.

The National Association of EMTs

The mission of the National Association of Emergency Medical Technicians, Inc. (NAEMT) is to be a professional representative organization that will receive and represent the views and opinions of prehospital care personnel and to thus influence the future advancement of Emergency Medical Services as an allied health profession. NAEMT will serve its professional membership through educational programs, liaison activities, development of national standards and reciprocity, and development of programs to benefit prehospital care personnel.

⊞ THE AMLS PROGRAM

Goals of the Course

The hands-on portion of the AMLS course gives each participant the ability to integrate the knowledge presented into a practical format for use in his or her current practice. While the course has a strong emphasis on the prehospital management of medical emergencies, each case study and hands-on practical lab station is altered to encompass registered nurses, respiratory therapists, physicians, residents, and other advanced level healthcare providers. The format and administrative policies set forth are those of the NAEMT.

The major goals of the AMLS course are to:

▶ Apply critical thinking skills in order to integrate pathophysiology with the assessment findings of a medical patient.

▶ Determine and differentiate between actual and potential patient problems.

▶ Advance the provider's ability to

— Conduct a competent medical examination that utilizes proper diagnostic skills, critical thinking, and interventions.

— Utilize problem-solving strategies in interventions and management alternatives.

— Communicate the pertinent findings and interventions to the receiving facility.

▶ Allow the provider to systematically work through a patient assessment and examine the possibilities and probabilities of differential diagnoses.

Provider Course

Advanced Medical Life Support (AMLS) is a two-day (16-hour) in-depth study of medical emergencies for the adult patient. The Provider Course emphasizes a pragmatic approach and systematic format to patient care. The course is designed to combine interactive case-study based lectures with hands-on physical assessments of patients. The participant will practice an assessment initially from a global perspective, taking into account the patient's environmental issues. This information will help the participant to formulate a general impression, determine the patient's status, and explore the possibilities of differential diagnoses. Using a systematic approach to obtain an initial assessment, vital signs, present-illness and past medical history, and a focused physical exam, the participant will begin to develop a rationale for the probabilities of differential diagnoses. The management of the patient will be determined by these probabilities.

Pre-course preparation is necessary for successful completion of the course. Participants must purchase a copy of the *Advanced Medical Life Support*, 2nd Ed., textbook and review the pre-course materials. The pretest must be completed prior to the first day of class.

Successful completion of the program consists of the following:

▶ Attendance at both days of the course

▶ A score of 76% or better on the written final exam

▶ Proficiency at the four assessment evaluation stations: Dyspnea/Respiratory Distress, Chest Pain (also includes Hypoperfusion), Abdominal Pain/GI Bleeding, and Altered Mental Status.

Upon successful completion, the basic and advanced participant will have received 16 hours of continuing education and will be awarded an Advanced Medical Life Support Provider certificate and wallet card. EMT-Basics will receive an Advanced Medical Life Support Basic Provider certificate and wallet card. Advanced providers will receive an Advanced Provider certificate and card. The continuing education credits are approved by the Continuing Education Coordinating Board of Emergency Medical Services (CECBEMS) and the NAEMT Education Accreditation Committee.

Because medicine is ever changing, periodic revisions and updates will be required as the scientific and medical fields uncover new advances and techniques. Therefore, the AMLS Provider, Instructor, and Affiliate Faculty recognition is valid for three years.

The Provider Course may compliment the medical emergency module of the paramedic course curriculum.

Instructor Course

The AMLS Instructor Course is designed to be a 4-hour course for those who have achieved an instructor-candidate potential when successfully completing an AMLS Provider Course with a posttest minimum score of 84% and a superior rating in evaluation stations. This course can be held following a provider course or as a stand-alone course. Upon completion of the course, the participant is considered an AMLS Instructor-Candidate. Instructor-Candidates must be monitored as they teach a Provider Course by Affiliate Faculty within one year of attending an instructor course in order to obtain an Instructor card. Affiliate Faculty award Instructor cards.

This course offers training to Instructor-Candidates that enables them to conduct provider and refresher courses using the AMLS philosophy and techniques and assists them in disseminating the course content. Individuals selected to attend this course are typically experienced instructors at the advanced healthcare level and coordinators and administrators with clinical skills and knowledge at an advanced level.

Refresher Course

The AMLS Refresher Course is designed to be an 4-hour course. It is offered to current AMLS providers who are nearing the expiration of their three-year recognition. The course incorporates case-based interactive lectures and evaluation stations.

Successful completion requires competency in the four evaluation stations: Altered Mental Status, Chest Pain (includes Hypoperfusion), Dyspnea/Respiratory Distress, and Abdominal Pain/GI Bleeding. In addition, a minimum score of 76% on the written exam must be achieved. An AMLS wallet card will be awarded by the Affiliate Faculty upon successful completion.

Instructor Update

The AMLS textbook, this Coordinator and Instructor Guide, and the accompanying CD-ROM will be reviewed and revised on a continuous basis. New information will be published as new science and trends unfold in our ever-changing medical field. Information regarding these changes will be forwarded to Instructors and Affiliate Faculty by memorandum, E-mail, electronically on new CD-ROMs, or by AMLS Instructor Update Workshops. The process will be determined as the need arises and at the guidance of NAEMT and the AMLS Executive Council. If deemed necessary, there will be a phase-in period during which the previous edition will still be available for those who have not attended an update workshop. Workshop update information will be distributed along with notification of effective dates for use of the new materials.

⊞ COURSE MATERIALS

The AMLS Text and Instructor Resources

The required textbook for this course is *Advanced Medical Life Support,* 2nd Ed., published by Brady/Prentice Hall. This textbook will serve as the primary resource throughout the course. It should be emphasized that each participant should purchase the textbook at least one month in advance of the course, to allow an opportunity to read through it. The textbook will give the participant a fundamental background that will be enhanced by the group practical sessions and by the introduction of critical thinking.

In order to ensure consistency in the delivery of material, no deviation from the prescribed NAEMT/AMLS course will be allowed. Utilization of the textbook is absolutely essential to successfully complete the course. It is the responsibility of the Course Coordinator to ensure that the textbook is obtained. The AMLS textbook can be ordered directly from Brady/Prentice Hall.

This *AMLS Coordinator and Instructor Guide* is an invaluable resource for the instructor who teaches the two-day AMLS course or implements the material in a medical emergencies didactic lecture series. The guide offers course objectives, case scenarios, and instructor's notes to accompany the slide program. The case scenarios in this guide are intended to be utilized with the appropriate assessment stations. These scenarios can be duplicated from the text for distribution to the appropriate instructor. Required equipment for each assessment station is minimal and is defined at the beginning of each scenario.

Pre-course materials such as handouts and pre- and post-tests can be obtained from the NAEMT office by the on-site coordinator when a course is registered. These materials are to be sent to participants along with the AMLS textbook 30 days prior to the course date. Duplication of all materials will be the responsibility of the hosting organization. It is of the utmost importance that the security of the post-tests be ensured to prevent any possibility of reproduction of the test itself.

The audio-visual PowerPoint slides for the Provider, Instructor, and Refresher courses are on CD-ROM. This CD-ROM is obtained from NAEMT when a course is registered. Only AMLS-recognized Course Coordinators and Affiliate Faculty will be awarded the CD-ROM. At this time, there is no fee for the CD-ROM. The CD-ROM may not be duplicated in its entirety for course instructors or be used within other programs. Its use is solely for the lecture presentations of the AMLS Provider, Instructor, and Refresher courses.

Educators may purchase additional AMLS audio-visual materials for utilization in other courses through Brady Publishing. These materials can be used in conjunction with the AMLS textbook.

⊞ COURSE FACULTY

AMLS Affiliate Faculty

The AMLS Affiliate Faculty are responsible for overseeing all the AMLS programs in their geographic area. The Affiliate Faculty are also responsible for making decisions, along with NAEMT, concerning possible changes in course material to meet local protocols, for ensuring that Course Coordinators are performing their jobs, and for acting as a direct extension of NAEMT for the AMLS course.

Qualifications needed for appointment to Affiliate Faculty include:

▶ Recognition as a monitored AMLS instructor by attendance at AMLS Provider and Instructor courses.

▶ Resume on file at the NAEMT office that indicates previous experience as Affiliate/Regional faculty for other continuing education courses, such as ACLS, PALS, PEPP, PPC, PHTLS, or BTLS.

▶ The time and ability to devote to monitoring and/or supervising area courses.

▶ Letter of recommendation from local Medical Director or AMLS Affiliate Faculty.

▶ Experience teaching and coordinating a minimum of one Provider Course with a satisfactory evaluation from AMLS Affiliate Faculty.

▶ The appropriate paperwork (stated above) is submitted to the AMLS Executive Council at the NAEMT office. The individual will then receive an AMLS Affiliate Faculty recognition wallet card. This recognition is valid for three years.

Job Description—The Affiliate Faculty are required to:

▶ Assist with curriculum development and implementation.

▶ Be available or on site during the course. Medical direction should also be accessible during the course.

▶ Teach and participate in a minimum of one course each year.

▶ Provide remediation in lieu of the Course Coordinator or Medical Director.

▶ Monitor Instructor-Candidates and ensure the appropriate forms (resumes and monitor form) are submitted with the post-course paperwork.

▶ Adhere to all NAEMT/AMLS standards to ensure course quality and integrity.

Course Coordinator

The Course Coordinator is responsible for overseeing the day-to-day operations of each individual course. This person is ultimately the key to the success of this course. The Course Coordinator is responsible for answering any questions that may arise, ensuring that proper station equipment is available and that live patients participate in all teaching and evaluation stations, and handling administrative duties for the course.

Qualifications—The Course Coordinator must have:

▶ Completed AMLS Provider and Instructor courses.

▶ Previous experience coordinating PHTLS, BTLS, ACLS, PALS, PPC, PEPP, etc.

▶ Access to the necessary equipment and facilities that are vital to carrying out a class.

Job Description—The Course Coordinator is required to:

▶ Compile all pre-course packets for participants, course registration, completed post-course material, and instructor-candidate evaluations.

▶ Ensure that all post-course paperwork is submitted to NAEMT within 30 days of the course completion. The post-course paperwork includes:

— Instructor monitoring forms

— Course evaluations

— Written exam grades

— Verification of competency in the evaluation stations

— Roster for participation in Provider/Instructor/Refresher Course

— In addition, a check payable to NAEMT for each participant. (There is a surcharge of $15/Provider Course participant, $10/Instructor Course participant, and $10/Refresher Course participant.)

▶ Adhere to all NAEMT/AMLS standards to ensure course security and integrity.

▶ Identify on the course application the on-site hosting organization.

▶ Coordinate and/or teach a minimum of one course per year.

AMLS Instructor

The AMLS Instructor is the core, or backbone, of the educational component of this course. The AMLS Instructor certification is valid for three years and requires that the instructor teaches a minimum of one course each year. Instructors should be utilized in their area of expertise. This should ensure a high level of expertise in all the different areas.

Qualifications—The AMLS Instructor must:

▶ Have completed an AMLS Provider Course and received an instructor potential rating. (An instructor potential rating is acquired by achieving an 84% or higher on the Provider Course written exam and a superior rating on one's performance in the teaching and evaluation stations.)

▶ Be monitored by an Affiliate Faculty member within one year of becoming an instructor.

▶ Have previous instructional experience in teaching PHTLS, ACLS, PALS, PPC, or equivalent advanced level courses.

▶ Have current status as an advanced healthcare professional/provider.

▶ Have successfully completed the Instructor and Provider Courses to be recognized as an Instructor-Candidate.

▶ Be monitored by Affiliate Faculty, lecturing and providing instruction in a Provider Course within one year of the Instructor Course. Once the instructor-candidate is monitored with a favorable rating by the Affiliate Faculty, the Affiliate Faculty will award the instructor card.

▶ Teach in at least one AMLS course per year.

Additional Requirements:

▶ All instructor-candidates must submit a curriculum vitae/resumé to the Course Coordinator/Affiliate Faculty for submission to the NAEMT office with post-course paperwork.

▶ Upon successfully completing the Instructor Course, candidates will be required to participate in the lecture and laboratory portions of an AMLS course.

Job Description—The AMLS Instructor is required to:

▶ Adhere to all NAEMT/AMLS standards to ensure course security and integrity.

▶ Maintain competency in all areas of AMLS.

▶ Complete the necessary documentation for the practical stations.

▶ Report any necessary information to the Course Coordinator or Affiliate Faculty member.

⊞ ADDITIONAL COURSE FACULTY

Additional course faculty are course members who are not necessarily AMLS instructors or providers, but do act as integral members of the AMLS team. These team members include Medical Director, Hosting Organization, Assessment Evaluators, and patients.

Medical Director

A Medical Director is a very important aspect of this course. The Medical Director will give guidance to faculty on the accuracy of information, provide insight into technical areas, and answer any questions that are brought to his or her attention. Additionally, the Medical Director should have some involvement in training, educating, or directing EMS providers in his or her area. This will allow the physician to be familiar with the current local standards/operational orders in prehospital emergency care. Each Medical Director needs to be approved by the region's Affiliate Faculty to ensure that the necessary requirements are met. The course Medical Director must be available during the course to answer questions and provide medical direction.

Qualifications—The Medical Director must be:

▶ A licensed practicing physician (MD or DO).

▶ Actively involved in prehospital emergency medicine or currently practice in a primary care area of medicine and have an interest in EMS.

Job Description—The Medical Director is required to:

▶ Ensure the accuracy of all medical-related information.

▶ Serve as a resource person, answering questions for faculty and participants.

▶ Act together with the Affiliate Faculty, Course Coordinator, and instructors to resolve any problems or conflicts during the course.

▶ Adhere to the NAEMT/AMLS course guidelines and standards.

Hosting Organization

The local Hosting Organization has many different roles and responsibilities that will need to be fulfilled in order for the course to be a success. The Hosting Organization is the on-site location of the course coordinator.

Responsibilities—The Hosting Organization must:

▶ Provide adequate facilities for the course, which include, but are not limited to, a lecture room with adequate seating for all participants, rooms to conduct practical examinations in, restroom facilities, adequate eating facilities located nearby, telephone, fax, and copy machine.

▶ Provide AMLS instructors, patients, and a Medical Director for the course.

▶ Work closely with local NAEMT and EMS representatives to advertise the course appropriately.

▶ Develop a working budget to allow for necessary expenses, such as bringing in out-of-town instructors and guest lecturers and providing for all of their travel expenses.

▶ Seek out and handle all administrative responsibilities necessary for the granting of continuing education hours where allowed.

Assessment Evaluator

Qualifications—The Assessment Evaluator must have:

▶ Active licensure, certification, and registration as a healthcare provider.

▶ Core knowledge of and skills proficiency in the specific area he or she is evaluating.

▶ Knowledge of prehospital emergency medicine.

Job Description—The Assessment Evaluator is required to:

▶ Fairly and accurately evaluate individual performance in patient assessment.

▶ Abide by NAEMT/AMLS course guidelines and standards.

Patients

All Provider Courses and Refresher Courses will need to have a minimum of 4 individuals who will serve as patients for the teaching and evaluation stations. This will enhance the learning process by allowing participants some "real-time" hands-on practice with the assessment skills. There should be a mixture of both male and female patients to compliment the scenarios.

Job Description—The Patient is required to:

▶ Accurately portray a patient with a specific set of pathophysiologic conditions.

▶ Interact with participants and the Assessment Evaluator as needed.

AMLS Provider

The AMLS Provider is one who has successfully completed the NAEMT/ AMLS course and has successfully passed both the cognitive and skills performance examinations in accordance with the NAEMT/AMLS standards. On successful completion, the AMLS Provider will be issued a certificate of completion that will be valid for three years. An AMLS Refresher Course will renew AMLS Provider recognition.

◫ PARTICIPANT PREREQUISITES

Because AMLS is an advanced course that assumes a previous working knowledge of medical emergencies, there are necessary prerequisites. Course participation is open to all providers: EMT-Paramedics (EMT-Ps), EMT-Intermediates (EMT-Is), EMT-Basics (EMT-Bs), and to Registered Nurses (RNs) or Physicians (MDs/DOs) with at least one year of clinical experience. **However, this is an advanced level course and, as such, the participant must be academically and clinically prepared for a rapid-paced and thought-provoking class.** This will ensure that participants have the base knowledge and experience on which the AMLS course will build. To successfully complete the course, the participant *must* read the AMLS textbook before the class and come to class prepared.

The second revision of the AMLS Instructor/Coordinator guideline now includes a separate written evaluation for EMT-Basic providers. This allows more inclusion of basic level providers. Evaluation scenarios may be evaluated for competency at the basic level. AMLS basic level provider certificates and cards should be awarded. Requests for basic level certificates and cards should be indicated on the course application form.

◫ COURSE SIZE

To maximize learning potential, class size is dependent on the instructor/ patient to participant ratio. For each practical station, the highest ratio of instructor/patient to participant allowed will be one instructor/one patient for every five participants. Smaller ratios allow participants to have more time to practice and review each scenario. The success of the course relies on application of the didactic material to the physical assessment.

◫ COURSE OUTLINES

The course outline has been developed to offer a proposed pattern for each course. The lecture content is specifically set to allow each instructor to build on concepts previously covered. This syllabus should be adhered to closely. At no time should a lecture be moved or shortened without previous acknowledgment of the Affiliate Faculty and NAEMT. The two-day proposed schedules are provided on the following pages. Schedule A includes the optional Airway Management scenario station.

AMLS Provider Course: Sample Schedule A

Schedule A (Optional Airway Management Scenario Station)

Day 1

0730   Registration

0800   Introduction, Course Overview

0815   Lecture: Assessment of the Medical Patient

0915   Break

0930   Lecture: Airway Management, Ventilation, and Oxygen Therapy

1030   Group Rotations: Assessment (Case 1) and Airway (Case 1)

1130   Lecture: Hypoperfusion (Shock)

1230   Lunch

1315   Group Rotations: Hypoperfusion (Cases 1 to 4)

1435   Lecture: Dyspnea, Respiratory Distress, or Respiratory Failure

1535   Lecture: Chest Pain

1635   Group Rotations: Dyspnea (Cases 1 and 2) and Chest Pain (Cases 1 and 2)

1800   Adjourn

Day 2

0800   Lecture: Altered Mental Status

0900   Lecture: Abdominal Pain/GI Bleeding

1000   Break

1015   Group Rotations: Altered Mental Status (Cases 1 and 2) and Abdominal Pain/GI Bleeding (Cases 1 and 2)

1135   Pretest Review

1200   Lunch

1245   Final Exam Rotations—Case 4 Evaluation Scenarios (4 topics: Dyspnea, Chest Pain, Altered Mental Status, and Abdominal Pain/GI Bleeding) and Written Exam

1545   Course Evaluation, Certificates/Cards Awarded

AMLS PROVIDER COURSE: SAMPLE SCHEDULE A

Group Rotations for 6–10 Participants

▶ Number of instructors: 2

▶ Group size: 3–5 participants per group

Day 1 *(with optional Airway Management Scenario)*

	1030–1100	**1100–1130**
Assessment (Case 1)	Group A	Group B
Airway (Case 1)	Group B	Group A

	1315-1355	**1355-1435**
Hypoperfusion (Cases 1 and 2)	Group A	Group B
Hypoperfusion (Cases 3 and 4)	Group B	Group A

	1635–1715	**1715–1755**
Dyspnea (Cases 1 and 2)	Group A	Group B
Chest Pain (Cases 1 and 2)	Group B	Group A

Day 2

	1015–1055	**1055–1135**
Altered Mental Status (Cases 1 and 2)	Group A	Group B
Abdominal Pain/GI Bleeding (Cases 1 and 2)	Group B	Group A

Final Exam Rotations for 6–10 Participants

▶ Number of instructors: 3–4

▶ Group size: 2–3 participants per group

▶ All evaluation stations are Case 4 scenarios

Day 2

	1245–1315	**1315–1345**	**1345–1415**	**1415–1445**	**1445–1515**	**1515–1545**
Group A	Written	Written	I	II	III	IV
Group B	Written	Written	II	III	IV	I
Group C	I	II	III	IV	Written	Written

Key: I = Dyspnea; II = Chest Pain; III = Altered Mental Status; IV = Abdominal Pain/GI Bleeding.

Group Rotations for 12–20 Participants

▶ Number of instructors: 4

▶ Group size: 3–5 participants per group

Day 1 *(with optional Airway Management Scenarios)*

	1030–1100	1100–1130		
Assessment (Case 1A)	Group A	Group C		
Assessment Case 1B)	Group B	Group D		
Airway (Case 1A)	Group C	Group A		
Airway (Case 1B)	Group D	Group B		
	1315–1335	**1335–1355**	**1355–1415**	**1415–1435**
Hypoperfusion (Case 1)	Group A	Group B	Group C	Group D
Hypoperfusion (Case 2)	Group B	Group C	Group D	Group A
Hypoperfusion (Case 3)	Group C	Group D	Group A	Group B
Hypoperfusion (Case 4)	Group D	Group A	Group B	Group C
	1635–1715	**1715–1755**		
Dyspnea (Cases 1A and 2A)	Group A	Group C		
Dyspnea (Cases 1B and 2B)	Group B	Group D		
Chest Pain (Cases 1A and 2A)	Group C	Group A		
Chest Pain (Cases 1B and 2B)	Group D	Group B		

Day 2

	1015–1055	1055–1135
Altered Mental Status (Cases 1A and 2A)	Group A	Group C
Altered Mental Status (Cases 1B and 2B)	Group B	Group D
Abdominal Pain/GI Bleeding (Cases 1A and 2A)	Group C	Group A
Abdominal Pain/GI Bleeding (Cases 1B and 2B)	Group D	Group B

Final Exam Rotations for 12–20 Participants

▶ Number of instructors: 4–7

▶ Group size: 2–3 participants per group

▶ All evaluation stations are Case 4 scenarios

Day 2

	1245–1315	1315–1345	1345–1415	1415–1445	1445–1515	1515–1545
Group A	Written	Written	I	II	III	IV
Group B	Written	Written	II	III	IV	I
Group C	I	II	III	IV	Written	Written
Group D	II	III	IV	I	Written	Written

Key: I = Dyspnea; II = Chest Pain; III = Altered Mental Status; IV = Abdominal Pain/GI Bleeding.

AMLS PROVIDER COURSE: SAMPLE SCHEDULE B

Day 1

0730   Registration

0800   Introduction, Course Overview

0810   Lecture: Assessment of the Medical Patient

0915   Break

0930   Lecture: Airway Management, Ventilation, and Oxygen Therapy

1030   Lecture: Hypoperfusion (Shock)

1130   Group Rotations: Assessment (Cases 1 and 2) and Hypoperfusion (Cases 1 and 2)

1230   Lunch

1315   Lecture: Chest Pain

1415   Break

1430   Lecture: Dyspnea, Respiratory Distress, Respiratory Failure

1530   Group Rotations: Dyspnea (Cases 1 and 2) and Chest Pain (Cases 1 and 2)

1630   Adjourn

Day 2

0800   Lecture: Altered Mental Status

0900   Break

0915   Lecture: Abdominal Pain/GI Bleeding

1015   Group Rotations: Altered Mental Status (Cases 1 and 2) and Abdominal Pain/GI Bleeding (Cases 1 and 2)

1115   Pretest Review

1200   Lunch

1245   Final Exam Rotations—Case 4 Evaluation Scenarios (4 topics: Chest Pain, Dyspnea, Altered Mental Status, and Abdominal Pain/GI Bleeding) and Written Exam

1600   Course Evaluation, Certificates/Cards Awarded

Group Rotations for 6–10 Participants

► Number of instructors: 2

► Group size: 3–5 participants per group

Day 1

	1130–1200	1200–1230
Assessment (Cases 1 and 2)	Group A	Group B
Hypoperfusion (Cases 1 and 2)	Group B	Group A

	1530–1600	1600–1630
Dyspnea (Cases 1 and 2)	Group A	Group B
Chest Pain (Cases 1 and 2)	Group B	Group A

Day 2

	1015–1045	1045–1115
Altered Mental Status (Cases 1 and 2)	Group A	Group B
Abdominal Pain/GI Bleeding (Cases 1 and 2)	Group B	Group A

Final Exam Rotations for 6–10 Participants

► Number of instructors: 3–4

► Group size: 2–3 participants per group

► All evaluation stations are Case 4 scenarios

Day 2

	1245–1315	1315–1345	1345–1415	1415–1445	1445–1515	1515–1545
Group A	Written	Written	I	II	III	IV
Group B	I	II	III	IV	Written	Written

Key: I = Chest Pain; II = Dyspnea; III = Altered Mental Status; IV = Abdominal Pain/GI Bleeding.

Group Rotations for 12–20 Participants

▶ Number of instructors: 4

▶ Group size: 3–5 participants per group

NOTE: Case numbering 1A, 1B, etc. indicates same case scenario being presented simultaneously at two different stations.

Day 1

	1130–1200	1200–1230
Assessment (Cases 1A and 2A)	Group A	Group C
Assessment (Cases 1B and 2B)	Group B	Group D
Hypoperfusion (Cases 1A and 2A)	Group C	Group A
Hypoperfusion (Cases 1B and 2B)	Group D	Group B

	1530–1600	1600–1630
Dyspnea (Cases 1A and 2A)	Group A	Group C
Dyspnea (Cases 1B and 2B)	Group B	Group D
Chest Pain (Cases 1A and 2A)	Group C	Group A
Chest Pain (Cases 1B and 2B)	Group D	Group B

Day 2

	1015–1045	1045–1115
Altered Mental Status (Cases 1A and 2A)	Group A	Group C
Altered Mental Status (Cases 1B and 2B)	Group B	Group D
Abdominal Pain/GI Bleeding (Cases 1A and 2A)	Group C	Group A
Abdominal Pain/GI Bleeding (Cases 1B and 2B)	Group D	Group B

Final Exam Rotations for 12–20 Participants

▶ Number of instructors: 4–7

▶ Group size: 2–3 participants per group

▶ All evaluation stations are Case 4 scenarios

Day 2

	1245–1315	1315–1345	1345–1415	1415–1445	1445–1515	1515–1545
Group A	Written	Written	I	II	III	IV
Group B	Written	Written	II	III	IV	I
Group C	I	II	III	IV	Written	Written
Group D	II	III	IV	I	Written	Written

Key: I = Chest Pain; II = Dyspnea; III = Altered Mental Status; IV = Abdominal Pain/GI Bleeding.

⊞ COURSE BUDGET

It is the responsibility of the Hosting Organization to collect all participant fees; course fees for the facility, equipment, and refreshments (if provided); and to pay for any instructor costs (if previously arranged). Usually, fees are low because the available facility is often donated (by the hospital, fire department, community college, etc.); necessary equipment is minimal and usually can be borrowed from local EMS agencies; and many instructors donate their time for the course. The NAEMT surcharge is $15.00 per person for the Provider Course, $10.00 per participant for the Instructor Course, and $10.00 per participant for the Refresher Course. The cost of the course depends on the cost of the above-named variables along with the surcharge fees. NAEMT/AMLS does not require submission of your course budget with pre-course paperwork.

When determining course cost, figure in the cost of the following:

- ▶ NAEMT surcharge
- ▶ Facility fee
- ▶ Instructor honoraria
- ▶ Patient honoraria
- ▶ Additional course faculty honoraria
- ▶ Textbooks
- ▶ Audiovisual expenses
- ▶ Printing cost—pre- and post-tests, course handouts, etc.
- ▶ Advertisements
- ▶ Postage for mailings
- ▶ Refreshments
- ▶ Additional materials

The cost for a complete course may be higher the first few times that you host it due to travel expenses for your faculty or the import of Instructors/Affiliate Faculty to your location. After that, the additional course costs, such as audiovisual expenses, etc., are usually minimal and the overall course costs are reduced. Many of the above costs may also be eliminated if the Hosting Organization can provide the facility, instructors, audiovisual equipment, and copying for the AMLS staff.

⊞ COURSE CERTIFICATES AND CARDS

On successful completion of the course, the Course Coordinator must send the appropriate course paperwork within 30 days to NAEMT. The AMLS certificates and wallet cards are sent to the Course Coordinator/Affiliate Faculty when a course is registered. Participants should be awarded the appropriate certificate and card upon successful completion of the course. The Course Coordinator or Affiliate Faculty has the responsibility of distributing them to all appropriate course participants at the completion of the course.

⊞ COURSE PAPERWORK

Course Application/Course Budget

A proposed course will need to be approved by NAEMT 60 days in advance. Within 30 days of the course, a confirmation letter with course materials will be sent to the Course Coordinator. This letter will confirm that the course has been approved and registered. All registered courses will be placed on the AMLS Website. The proposed course application should include the:

▶ Name of the Hosting Organization

▶ Names of the Course Coordinator, Affiliate Faculty, instructors, and Medical Director

▶ Location and time frame of the course

▶ Agenda with AMLS instructor assignments

▶ Anticipated number of participants

NAEMT will review the proposed application for approval and registration. Upon approval a national course number will be issued and the appropriate pre-course materials will be forwarded to the Course Coordinator. Pre-course materials include, but are not limited to:

▶ Pretest

▶ Pretest annotated answer sheet

▶ Post-test I and II

▶ Test answer sheet

▶ Post-test I and II annotated answer sheet

▶ Assessment handout

▶ Math calculation handout

▶ NAEMT membership application

Participant Application

The participant application must be filled out by each participant. One copy of the application must be sent to the AMLS Executive Office and another to the Affiliate Faculty who is supervising the course. The participant's application and NAEMT surcharge must be sent to NAEMT before the post-course deadline and will become a permanent record at that office.

Course Rosters

The course roster will include all pertinent information about each participant, including the participant's name, address, telephone number, written evaluation score, and whether the participant passed or failed the evaluation stations. The roster needs to be signed by the Course Coordinator, the Affiliate Faculty, and the Medical Director. Hard copies of the information can be forwarded with the post-course paperwork or sent electronically by disk or E-mail. The E-mail address is AMLS@NAEMT.org.

Course Evaluations

Each participant will be required to fill out a course evaluation. Course evaluations should be submitted for Provider, Instructor, and Refresher courses. You may utilize a summary format to submit the scores and comments to NAEMT along with other post-course paperwork. This may also be sent electronically by disk or E-mail.

Instructor Evaluations

Instructor evaluations may be completed by participants as deemed appropriate by the Course Coordinator, Affiliate Faculty, and Medical Director. Each instructor should be given the opportunity to review these evaluations. These evaluations do not need to be forwarded to NAEMT with the post-course paperwork unless the Course Coordinator, Affiliate Faculty, or Medical Director deem appropriate.

⊞ INTERNATIONAL AMLS

Prior to the introduction of AMLS to another nation, several requirements must be achieved. On-site medical direction must be established and a core of AMLS instructors from the host country must be trained in the United States. It is preferred that the nation have an active PHTLS Program in place.

It is also preferred that the potential instructors, Course Coordinators, Affiliate Faculty, and Medical Directors travel to the United States and attend AMLS Provider and Instructor courses. The AMLS Provider and Instructor courses must be at an AMLS Executive Council approved site. This process will ensure the sponsors obtain insight on how the courses are organized. In this format, the AMLS Chairperson and/or designated committee faculty is able to assist with lectures and practical skills stations during the inaugural course.

Once a host country has signed the Memorandum of Understanding (MOU) with NAEMT and several AMLS instructors have been trained, dates are set for the country's inaugural AMLS course. Typically a 3-day Provider/Instructor course and a subsequent 2-day Provider course is scheduled. Participants for the Provider/Instructor courses are selected by the host country.

It is preferred to have the National Chairperson(s) and the AMLS Executive Committee Medical Director assist with the course. Upon completion of the inaugural Provider/Instructor course there is a one-day break. Following the one-day break, the new instructors are monitored by the United States faculty.

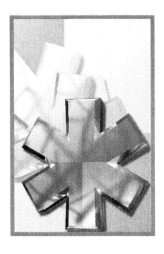

VII. ADVANCED MEDICAL LIFE SUPPORT COURSE FORMS

⊞ COURSE FORMS

The following forms are provided:

- ▶ NAEMT Advance Medical Life Support Course Application
- ▶ Advance Medical Life Support Course Budget
- ▶ Advance Medical Life Support Participant Application
- ▶ Advance Medical Life Support Course Roster
- ▶ Advance Medical Life Support Course Evaluation Form
- ▶ Advance Medical Life Support Instructor Evaluation Form
- ▶ Advance Medical Life Support Instructor-Candidate Monitoring Form
- ▶ Advance Medical Life Support Participant Final Evaluation Form
- ▶ NAEMT Advance Medical Life Support Graduation Pin Order Form
- ▶ Advance Medical Life Support Participant Exam Answer Sheet

NAEMT ADVANCED MEDICAL LIFE SUPPORT
COURSE APPLICATION*

Send to: The National Association of EMTs, AMLS Office, 408 Monroe Street, Clinton, MS 39056

I. Sponsor Information

A. Local Hosting Organization: _____

Address: _____

Phone: _____

B. Proposed Course Coordinator/Title: _____

Address: _____

Phone: (   ) _____ Ext: _____ E-mail: _____

C. Proposed Affiliate Faculty: _____

Address: _____

Phone: (   ) _____ Ext: _____ E-mail: _____

D. Proposed Course Medical Director: _____

Background: _____

ATLS Instructor? ☐ Yes ☐ No

Address: _____

Phone: (   ) _____ Ext: _____ E-mail: _____

II. National Course Number: _____ State Course Number: _____

A. Facility/On-site Location: _____

Address: _____

Contact Person/Phone: _____ (   ) _____

B. Proposed Course Dates: Start Date: _____ End Date: _____

C. Anticipated participant enrollment:

☐ Provider Course: Advanced Providers _____ Basic Providers _____

☐ Refresher Course: Advanced Providers _____ Basic Providers _____

☐ Instructor Course: Advanced Providers _____

D. Attach proposed course agenda with AMLS instructor assignments.

E. NAEMT CD-ROM needed? ☐ Yes ☐ No

F. We agree that the NAEMT regional faculty member on-site is the final authority on the conduct of the course and must be consulted in writing for approval before any alterations in schedule, etc. may be made.

| _____ | _____ |
| Date | Responsible Officer of Host Organization |

| _____ | _____ |
| Date | Proposed Course Coordinator |

| _____ | _____ |
| Date | Proposed Course Medical Director |

*NOTE: This form must be received by Affiliate Faculty 60 days in advance of proposed course dates.

ADVANCE MEDICAL LIFE SUPPORT
COURSE BUDGET

Course date(s): _____   Sponsor: _____

Submitted by: _____   Date: _____

EXPENSES

Personnel

Lecturers		
Skill station instructors		
Patients/moulage		
Secretarial support		
Other:		

Affiliate Faculty (as applicable)

Travel		
Lodging		
Meals		

Facilities

Facility charge		
Meals		
Refreshments		
Other:		

Materials, Equipment, and Supplies

Equipment rental		
Supplies		
Printing/duplication		
Brochures		
Postage		
Textbooks		
Other:		

NAEMT Surcharge

Provider: $15 × _____		
Instructor: $10 × _____		
Refresher: $10 × _____		

REVENUES

Tuition fee $ _____ × _____ participants		
Textbooks sold		
Meals fee (if charged)		
Other:		

TOTAL EXPENSES _____

TOTAL REVENUES _____

NET _____

Advance Medical Life Support
Participant Application

Name: _____

Address: _____

City: _____ State: _____ Zip: _____

Home Phone: _____ Work Phone: _____

E-mail: _____

Occupation: _____

Level of Healthcare Provider: _____

License/Certification No. and Expiration: _____

Course Type: ☐ Provider ☐ Refresher ☐ Instructor

Course Fee Attached: $ _____

IMPORTANT: A copy of your certification/licensure (front and back) along with payment in full must be received before the enrollment deadline.

ADVANCED MEDICAL LIFE SUPPORT COURSE ROSTER

Course Type: ☐ Provider ☐ Refresher ☐ Instructor National Course No.: _____

Course Coordinator: _____ Affiliate Faculty: _____ Medical Director: _____

Course Dates: _____ Location: _____

Participant Name	Participant Address	Phone Number	Provider Level (B, I, P, RN)	Written Exam Score	Evaluation Stations (P/F)	Current NAEMT (Y/N)	Course Completion (P/F)

_____
Course Coordinator's Signature

_____
Affiliate Faculty's Signature

_____
Medical Director's Signature

Advanced Medical Life Support Course Roster (Continued)

National Course No.: _____

Participant Name	Participant Address	Phone Number	Provider Level (B, I, P, RN)	Written Exam Score	Evaluation Stations (P/F)	Current NAEMT (Y/N)	Course Completion (P/F)

Advance Medical Life Support
Course Evaluation Form

Course Location: _____

Course Date(s): _____ Course Type: ☐ Provider ☐ Refresher ☐ Instructor

Please rate the following aspects of the course. The following scale will be utilized:

1—Excellent
2—Good
3—Fair
4—Adequate

1) Overall evaluation of the course   1   2   3   4

2) Overall presentation of lecture material   1   2   3   4

3) Overall knowledge of course faculty   1   2   3   4

4) Overall rating of the facility   1   2   3   4

5) Overall rating of the audiovisual material   1   2   3   4

6) How will you integrate or utilize the information presented in this course?

_____

_____

_____

7) What part of this course did you like best?

_____

_____

_____

8) What part of this course did you like least?

_____

_____

_____

9) Additional comments:

_____

_____

_____

_____

_____

_____

_____

ADVANCE MEDICAL LIFE SUPPORT
INSTRUCTOR EVALUATION FORM

Course Location: _____

Course Date(s): _____ Course Type: ☐ Provider ☐ Refresher ☐ Instructor

Lecture Topic: _____ Teaching/Testing Station: _____

Please rate the following aspects of the presenter and his or her presentation.
The following scale will be utilized:

1—Excellent
2—Good
3—Fair
4—Adequate

1) Presenter's ability to keep the audience's attention   1   2   3   4

2) Presenter's knowledge of lecture material   1   2   3   4

3) Presenter's ability to maintain the time schedule   1   2   3   4

4) Presenter's ability to integrate course material with practical application   1   2   3   4

5) Presenter's use of the audiovisual material   1   2   3   4

6) How will you integrate or utilize the information presented in this lecture?

_____
_____
_____

7) What part of this lecture did you like best?

_____
_____
_____

8) What part of this lecture did you like least?

_____
_____
_____

9) Additional comments:

_____
_____
_____
_____
_____

Advanced Medical Life Support
Instructor-Candidate Monitoring Form

Instructor-Candidate Name: _____

Provider Course Date: _____ Instructor Course Date: _____

Affiliate Faculty Monitor Name: _____

Lecture	Satisfactory	Unsatisfactory
Presents lecture in a logical, concise, sequential fashion		
Is familiar with the A/V slide content		
Emphasizes critical thinking skills and the field thinking process in the lecture		
Emphasizes "what's different" when comparing pathophysiology, signs and symptoms on tables within the lecture. For example: auscultating breath sounds in determining causes of shock		
Maintains the participants' attention: — Varies pace, uses clear transitions — Uses questions appropriately — Has good voice, eye contact, and gestures — Moves purposefully — Does not read — Uses correct vocabulary and pronunciation		
Summarizes important points in the lecture and upon conclusion		
Uses appropriate examples to illustrate important points		
Answers questions in a supportive manner		
Completes the lecture on time		

Comments on lecture presentation: _____

_____

_____

_____

Instructor Attitude and Role	Satisfactory	Unsatisfactory
Attends faculty meetings		
Attends other lectures within the course		
Enhances the quality of the course		
Demonstrates support for the AMLS program		

Comments: _____

_____

_____

_____

Instructor-Candidate Name: _____

Provider Course Date: _____ Instructor Course Date: _____

Affiliate Faculty Monitor Name: _____

Group Case Scenario Stations	Satisfactory	Unsatisfactory
Prepares scenario's patient appropriately		
Presents scenario clearly and concisely		
Organizes equipment appropriately		
Allows team leader and team interaction to proceed without assistance		
Enhances critical thinking/field thinking process by intermittently asking about: — Initial impression and differential diagnoses — Initial plan — Initial assessment and resuscitation vs. gathering history first — Re-evaluation of impression and plan		
Allows team to lead discussion of each case and the processes used to manage the patient		
Summarizes topic of scenario and important points from lecture		

Comments on scenario presentation: _____

_____

_____

_____

Recommendation:

☐ Satisfactory

☐ Unsatisfactory. I recommend remediation and re-monitoring for possible future role
as an AMLS Instructor.

☐ Unsatisfactory. I recommend that this Candidate not be allowed to proceed as an AMLS Instructor.

Signature of Affiliate Faculty Monitor: _____ Date: _____

Date sent to AMLS Office: _____

Copy in File: _____

ADVANCED MEDICAL LIFE SUPPORT
PARTICIPANT FINAL EVALUATION FORM

Team Leader: _____ Scenario Number: _____

Evaluator: _____ Beginning Time: _____ Ending Time: _____

Task	Completed YES	NO	Comments Regarding Deficiencies
Scene Safety			
Initial Impression			
Initial Assessment			
Mental Status			
Airway			
Breathing			
Circulation			
Disability			
Focused History (SAMPLE)			
Signs and Symptoms			
Allergies			
Medications			
Past Medical History			
Last Oral Intake			
Events Preceding			
OPQRST			
Onset			
Palliation/Provocation			
Quality			
Radiation			
Severity			
Time			
Vital Signs			
Respirations			
Pulse			
Blood Pressure			
Temperature			
Pulse Oximetry			
Focused Secondary			
Differential Diagnosis			
Appropriate Treatment			

Critical Criteria

The following areas have been identified as critical criteria. As such, if any item below is checked, the participant needs to repeat the station. Please document any rationale concerning the area checked in the notation section below.

- ☐ Body substance isolation not performed
- ☐ Scene was not determined to be safe
- ☐ Initial assessment not performed or performed in an inadequate manner
- ☐ Failure to adequately maintain Airway, Breathing, or Circulation at any time throughout the scenario
- ☐ Inability to establish stability vs. instability/life threat vs. non-life threat
- ☐ Focused history not performed or performed before initiation of life-saving measures
- ☐ Inappropriate treatment performed
- ☐ Appropriate treatment performed but in an untimely fashion
- ☐ Failure to complete the assessment in a timely manner

Additional Comments: _____ _____
_____
_____
_____

ADVANCE MEDICAL LIFE SUPPORT
GRADUATION PIN ORDER FORM

CONGRATULATIONS! You have earned the privilege to display the AMLS pin. The National Association of Emergency Medical Technicians is pleased to offer this distinctive pin. In order that you may receive your pin in a timely manner, the following information is necessary:

1) Please complete the information below.

2) Indicate the number of pins you desire.

3) Include a check, cashier's check, or money order (please, no cash through the mail) payable to NAEMT.

4) All taxes and shipping and handling charges are included in the $5.00 charge for each pin.

5) Return this form, payment, and a copy of your AMLS certificate to the address below. Please allow approximately two weeks for delivery.

ADVANCED MEDICAL LIFE SUPPORT PIN . . . . *$5.00 ea.*

Number of pins desired _____ $\times$ $5.00 = _____

PLEASE PRINT:

Name: _____

Address: _____

City: _____ State: _____ Zip: _____

Phone: (   ) _____ Ext: _____ E-mail: _____

NAEMT/AMLS

408 Monroe Street

Clinton, MS 39056

ADVANCE MEDICAL LIFE SUPPORT
PARTICIPANT EXAM ANSWER SHEET

Participant Name: _____ Date: _____ Score: _____

Course Location: _____

Circle and Mark One: BLS or ALS Pretest _____ BLS or ALS Post-test I _____ BLS or ALS Post-test II _____

1.	A	B	C	D		26.	A	B	C	D
2.	A	B	C	D		27.	A	B	C	D
3.	A	B	C	D		28.	A	B	C	D
4.	A	B	C	D		29.	A	B	C	D
5.	A	B	C	D		30.	A	B	C	D
6.	A	B	C	D		31.	A	B	C	D
7.	A	B	C	D		32.	A	B	C	D
8.	A	B	C	D		33.	A	B	C	D
9.	A	B	C	D		34.	A	B	C	D
10.	A	B	C	D		35.	A	B	C	D
11.	A	B	C	D		36.	A	B	C	D
12.	A	B	C	D		37.	A	B	C	D
13.	A	B	C	D		38.	A	B	C	D
14.	A	B	C	D		39.	A	B	C	D
15.	A	B	C	D		40.	A	B	C	D
16.	A	B	C	D		41.	A	B	C	D
17.	A	B	C	D		42.	A	B	C	D
18.	A	B	C	D		43.	A	B	C	D
19.	A	B	C	D		44.	A	B	C	D
20.	A	B	C	D		45.	A	B	C	D
21.	A	B	C	D		46.	A	B	C	D
22.	A	B	C	D		47.	A	B	C	D
23.	A	B	C	D		48.	A	B	C	D
24.	A	B	C	D		49.	A	B	C	D
25.	A	B	C	D		50.	A	B	C	D